The Menopause Transition in a Relationship Context

Drawing on a small-scale longitudinal study of midlife women tracking their menstrual cycles within the context of their lives as a whole over a 20-year period, this insightful book documents general health, family, and life situation changes and continuities for the participants. At once a research report, a memoir, and a commentary, this book uses rich interview data to explore the complexity of living beings consistently over time. Told through the women's own voices, it shows diversity and commonality of experience and develops a new method of assessing interlocking variables, the Multiple Continuum Assessment, which represents the complexity of life as fluid, systemic, and opportunistic.

This book makes the case that menopause is more than a collection of signs and symptoms. Women and their families experience continual change as a matter of fact. Overwhelmingly, they transact transitions with interest, survive challenges, develop new skills and resources, and come out on the other side. It concludes with recommendations for women, health care professionals, and researchers.

This innovative work is suitable for practitioners and academics with an interest in women's health, women's and gender studies, aging and health care, menopause transition, and family systems research, as well as women themselves.

Nomi Redding is a retired psychotherapist/clinical social worker and researcher based in Lawrence, Kansas, USA.

The Menopause Transition in a Relationship Context

Voices and Choices at Midlife, 1991–2012

Nomi Redding

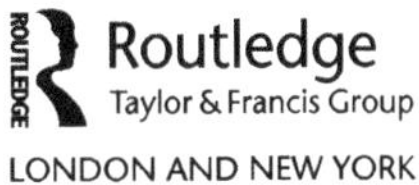

Routledge
Taylor & Francis Group

LONDON AND NEW YORK

First published 2025
by Routledge
4 Park Square, Milton Park, Abingdon, Oxon OX14 4RN

and by Routledge
605 Third Avenue, New York, NY 10158

Routledge is an imprint of the Taylor & Francis Group, an informa business

British Library Cataloguing-in-Publication Data
A catalogue record for this book is available from the British Library

ISBN: 978-1-032-89018-0 (hbk)
ISBN: 978-1-032-99075-0 (pbk)
ISBN: 978-1-003-54083-0 (ebk)

DOI: 10.4324/9781003540830

Typeset in Times New Roman
by codeMantra

"To All the Women Who Raised Their Voices"

Contents

Preface

In 1991, the first of the Baby Boomers were turning 45, and menopause burst into public view and personal conversations as a hot topic. Accidentally and on purpose, I happened into a research study that would occupy me for 30 years and is yet.

It was no accident that I, who grew up in a house of science and service and practiced social work from a clinical theory grounded in natural science, would do research. But beginning a study intended as a two-year pilot project, I never imagined it would last for 20 years, mirror events in my own life, and introduce me to colleagues and contacts the world over.

Family Roots

My father, the oldest of two sons born to immigrant parents, came out of WWII with the GI bill and the ambition to finish his bachelor's degree followed immediately by graduate work. Earning his doctorate in parasitology when I was not yet three years old, he went into university teaching and basic research. He embodied the qualities of the researcher he taught his students: (1) curiosity and the ability to organize curiosity; (2) drive and stubborn determination; and (3) objectivity and honesty.

My mother, the youngest of five, whose own immigrant parents were older than my father's, did not have the opportunity for higher education, but supported my father's career in multiple ways while also reading voraciously in a wide variety of fields. She gravitated toward psychology as a way to make sense of her own family and the world. She served as a listening ear for neighbors and friends alike.

While my dad's interests took him into the woods, the lab, and the classroom, my mom functioned in the world of people and their relationships. Provided the framework for doing research from him and the lens for humans from her, I gained a compelling base from which to develop my own interests.

My younger sister and I went into service careers, she in nursing following my mother's aspiration, I in social work, my godmother's field. After working seven years post-master's in medical settings, I pivoted to clinical work in a private practice where I stayed 30 years. In my first year of practice, I began advanced training from a family systems perspective compatible with my roots. Those of us studying Bowen Theory were encouraged to understand our own families as natural systems and to pursue research projects following Dr. Bowen's example integrating knowledge from the natural sciences with family theory. I gravitated toward reproductive functioning as my area of study which fit with my family history and personal experience with endometriosis and infant loss. Happily, by the time of the first interviews in the research project, my high school sweetheart and I were in our 24th year of marriage and parenting our then ten-year-old daughter.

Professional Roots: Models for Research

Murray Bowen, MD, Bowen Family Systems Theory and Therapy

Originally from Tennessee, Dr. Bowen served in WWII assuming he would go on to specialize in surgery but came out convinced there was a greater need for effective advances in mental health. While studying at the Menninger Foundation in Topeka, KS, he read everything in the library to do with science and its assumptions. He developed the hypothesis that human problems were based on what we share with other life forms, not where we differ. Moving on to the National Institutes of Health (NIH) in Washington, DC, he designed a research project hospitalizing families who had a member diagnosed with schizophrenia. By the time he left NIH for Georgetown University, the eight basic concepts of his multigenerational family systems theory were in place and he had evidence they applied universally. Viewing families as functional units and emotional processes as fundamental to functioning, he concluded that the lives of individuals must be understood within the context of their relationship systems.

From September 1982 until his death in October 1990, I had the good fortune to read written work by Dr. Bowen, hear him speak in person at professional meetings, and consult with him personally at his home office in Bethesda, MD. During our first meeting, he commented, "Being yourself is your birthright," possibly the most freeing statement I had ever heard. When I returned to Lawrence and shared it with my mother she responded, "Oh-like fingerprints." My second meeting with him came after I had written my first papers reviewing the literature on menopause. He likened that to his library study at Menninger. Encouraging me to continue, he was less concerned with the educational degrees I held than the effort to diligently conduct systematic research saying, "Make yourself appear useful."

Alan Treloar, PhD, The Menstrual and Reproductive Health Program (MRH, now the TREMIN Research Program on Women's Health)

Dr. Treloar emigrated from Australia to the United States in 1926 to earn a PhD in agricultural biochemistry at the University of Minnesota. Once there, he met "this newfangled stuff called statistics" and instead pursued the field of biometry. Carrying out a study of infant development, he doubted the prevailing assumption of menstrual regularity as a variable to estimate the duration of pregnancy and decided to investigate. Beginning in 1934, he and his colleagues enrolled women students in the Menstrual and Reproductive Health (MRH) program collecting prospective data of their menstrual cycles. He ultimately concluded that regularity as applied to the menstrual cycle was a vague term and should not be taken literally to mean without variation. Decades after its inception, the Tremin Trust Project would be described as "The World's Oldest Ongoing Study of Menstruation and Women's Health."

Impressed by reading his work found during my literature review, I attempted to contact Dr. Treloar to learn more. I tracked him from the University of Minnesota to a former colleague then in Chapel Hill, North Carolina, and finally to the University of Arizona. Using his last known address from a listing in American Men and Women of Science, my husband and I made a side trip to Sun City during a spring break visit with his parents, then retired "snowbirds" in Mesa City. We learned Dr. Treloar no longer lived at the address I had found. However, I was fortunate to have a wonderful conversation with his former next-door neighbor. She well remembered the MRH project files in his garage "all those punch cards" and gave me contact information of his daughter in California who then kindly answered my follow-up letter. Explaining the MRH project was now directed by Dr. Ann Voda at the School of Nursing, University of Utah, she wrote, "I'm sure my father would have greatly appreciated your interest in his research. Unfortunately, his mental faculties have declined markedly in the past year or two." Serendipitously, I was to meet Ann at my first professional menstrual cycle research meeting in Seattle two months later. Dr. Treloar died the year after Dr. Bowen in November 1991.

Dr. Bowen and Dr. Treloar were trailblazers in their respective fields, original thinkers not afraid to question prevailing dogma and motivated for long-term effort and exploration. Together their research provided models that informed the design for this study.

References

Rakow, C.M. (2023). *Making sense of human life: Murray Bowen's determined effort toward family systems theory*. New York and London: Routledge. https://doi.org/10.4324/9781003027287

Voda, A., Morgan, J., Root, J., & Smith, K. (1990). The Tremin Trust: An intergenerational research program on events associated with women's menstrual and reproductive lives. An update: 1990. The Tremin Trust Research Program.

Acknowledgments

In addition to the research of Dr. Bowen and Dr. Treloar whose work served as the pillars for the project design, I have been consistently encouraged and inspired by multiple researchers in both the family and menstrual cycle research fields. From my first meeting at the Society for Menstrual Cycle Research in 1991, I was warmly welcomed into an intergenerational, international group, whose global reach has only increased in ensuing decades. While topics, methods, and concerns may change, the mentoring commitment of those with experience to those whose work is up and coming is consistent to this day. I am happy in my turn to encourage young researchers who may never have considered the possibility of longitudinal work.

My colleagues in family systems have provided an excellent sounding base for my efforts to become clearer about my functioning in my own family and initiate and maintain this research. The initial aim of Dr. Bowen to move study of the human being toward the natural sciences is alive and well. Systems biology is but one interesting partner in addressing the complexity of living beings and their interrelationships with their environments. I look forward to the continuing conversation with dedicated researchers the world over, particularly as the means of electronic communication have multiplied and become increasingly accessible.

My own multigenerational family continues to be a source of support and inspiration. My parents left legacies carried through to the continuing generations of my sister and myself, our children, and grandchildren. My dear husband, partner extraordinaire, suggested how I could arrange my clinical schedule to free a day that was devoted to pure research. His patience as I pile papers in any number of rooms while working on projects is never assumed but always appreciated. It has been a blessing to witness our daughter establish her own place in the world as another successful solo practitioner while raising two eager, able, and curious children.

My women friends and I traveled through menopause together, each with our own story, but happy to share the tips, quirks, and challenges of midlife. There is something necessary and fundamental about the support of "chosen" family that softens some of the hardest times and enhances the most joyous.

And finally, to the continued grounding of mindfulness meditation, which my mother brought to me in 1993 and which practice I share with Plum Village communities all over the world. I am grateful for the peace and possibility of any given moment.

Bringing this project to resolution has been a first for me many times at many levels. I am grateful for the learning, for the kind cooperation of so many others, and most recently, from the fine publishing team at Taylor & Francis/Routledge. I appreciate each and every one of you.

Abbreviations and Acronyms

D & C	Dilation and curettage is a procedure to remove tissue from inside the uterus.
ENT	It is the medical abbreviation for ear, nose, and throat, referring to a medical specialty also known as otolaryngology focusing on diseases of the head and neck.
ER	Emergency room in a medical setting.
FDR	Franklin Delano Roosevelt is the 32nd President of the United States who served from 1933 until his death in 1945.
FMP	Final menstrual period.
FSH	Follicle-stimulating hormone is a hormone that regulates sexual development and reproduction in both men and women and is produced by the anterior pituitary gland. Levels may vary by age and sex and can be measured with a blood test.
HT	Hormone therapy, also known as menopausal hormone therapy (MHT) or hormone replacement therapy (HRT), is a treatment that uses hormones advertised to help relieve symptoms of menopause and address long-term biological changes. The most common prescriptions during the research study were for Premphase and Prempro marketed by Pfizer, estrogen plus progestin for women with a uterus for the treatment of moderate to severe vasomotor symptoms due to menopause, moderate to severe vulvar and vaginal atrophy due to menopause, and/or prevention of osteoporosis. Prescribed differently: One Prempro tablet taken orally once daily; one Premphase tablet taken orally on days 1 through 24, and another tablet taken orally on days 15 to 28.
ICU	Intensive Care Unit in a medical facility.
IUD	Intrauterine Device
KU	The University of Kansas, USA.
MAPS	Menopausal Adaptation Process Study.

MD   Doctor of Medicine.

MRH   Menstrual and Reproductive Health is the initial name of the longitudinal study of the menstrual cycle initiated by Dr. Treloar and colleagues at the University of Minnesota in 1934.

MWMHP   The Melbourne Women's Midlife Health Project.

NAMS   North American Menopause Society.

NASW   National Association of Social Workers.

OB/GYN   Obstetrician gynecologist is a medical specialty combining two disciplines and includes the care of a woman's reproductive organs and health, as well as the treatment of pregnant women.

PhD   Doctor of Philosophy.

PMS   Premenstrual syndrome is characterized as a group of physical and/or psychological symptoms that can occur before a woman's period with symptoms varying from mild to severe.

PMZ   Postmenopause zest is a term attributed to Margaret Mead and is used to highlight well-being in the postmenopause years.

SMCR   Society for Menstrual Cycle Research.

SMWHS   The Seattle Midlife Women's Health Study.

STRAW   Stage of Reproductive Aging Workshop.

SWAN   The Study of Women's Health Across the Nation.

TREMIN   aka the Tremin Trust; it is a program based on the menstrual cycle research of Dr. Alan Treloar and associates.

WHI   Women's Health Initiative is a long-term study focused on the prevention of heart disease, cancer, and osteoporosis in postmenopausal women.

Part 1

The Project

The Menopause Transition in a Relationship Context captures the journeys of a group of women through midlife in their own words, as they tracked their waning and variant menstrual cycles and annually updated general health, family, and life situation information. This book also reports the author's own journey as the principal investigator for the Menopausal Adaptation Process Study (MAPS), walking the same path as another midlife woman.

DOI: 10.4324/9781003540830-1

1 Introduction

In the spring of 1989 when I was 41, I noticed my menstrual cycles becoming a bit irregular. It was a very subtle change, but I was a woman whose cycle had traditionally been so predictable that in undergraduate school I knew in which class my period would start and could come prepared. The first shift from my traditional pattern was a somewhat shorter interval, the flows arriving closer together. The same spring I developed a new physical symptom. Having experienced allergies most of my life, I suddenly observed a heaviness in my chest about a mile into my morning walk. This was diagnosed as exercise asthma, helped by using an inhaler before I set out. The combination of the change in cycle plus a new symptom seemingly unrelated to any current stresses made me wonder about menopause.

As a good family therapist steeped in theory would do, I took the idea to my mother and asked her about the change of life experience for women in our branch of the family. For herself, she remembered years in her late 40s and early 50s of frequent heavy periods but thought of that as just one more thing she had to cope with at the time my father's health was deteriorating, ending with his death from cancer when she was 55. She didn't recall having hot flashes or menopausal symptoms other than the changes in interval and flow, and she had not done anything specifically to get her through.

With regard to my grandmothers, my mother recalled my father's mother having experienced a seemingly smooth transition in which she welcomed the end to the risk of pregnancy. For her own mother, my mother reported a much more dramatic story in which the mood of the whole family rode up and down according to whether Grandma had had "her shot," which cost $1 if she went to the doctor's office and $2 if he came to the house. My mother's mother and all three of my mother's older sisters eventually had hysterectomies. My father had no sisters so there were no paternal aunts to compare. This diversity of experience just within my own family made me curious to investigate further.

The glimmer of an idea for this research project came with the initial review of the literature in which I simply wished to learn more about menopause. Early on I spoke with a reference librarian at the Menninger Foundation, then

DOI: 10.4324/9781003540830-2

located in my neighboring community of Topeka, KS. She listened carefully, then told me, "You're going to have to limit your topic." I thought to myself, "That's exactly what I don't want to do."

Literature Review 1989–1991

Between the spring of 1989 and the fall of 1991, I read about menopause, including popular accounts, mainstream media, and self-help books, as well as scholarly information from the fields of biology, medicine, epidemiology, psychology, sociology, anthropology, and evolution, coming away with more questions than answers. Reviewing the literature gave me knowledge about the subject, and the multiple ways it had been studied and was regarded. Researchers treated menopause as both a physiological marker (the end to menstruation) and a transition in the family (the end to reproduction for a generation). It seemed that the researcher's perspective framed observations and influenced conclusions and recommendations. Debates on whether menopause was a hormonal, psychological, or sociocultural phenomenon did not interest me particularly, as I assumed it was all of these. Whatever was going to happen to me in this era, I knew it was going to occur in one body, within my ongoing life situation and relationships.

I was interested to learn the facts of menopause as women experienced them, leading their lives as usual. Alan Treloar's longitudinal research stood out as a model for observing menstrual facts over time without intervening in them. I was aware through my training and study of Bowen's theory that the multigenerational family diagram is an excellent tool for charting the life history of a relationship system. It seemed to me that Dr. Treloar's method of studying the menstrual cycle could be joined with Dr. Bowen's approach to studying families to learn about the menopause transition from women as they lived it.

I imagined doing a longitudinal study beginning with women in their 30s and following them until nearly age 60, tracking both menstrual cycle and family facts. Between my first trip to the library and beginning to enroll participants in the fall of 1991, I continued to read and talk with people about menopause. I joined the North American Menopause Society (NAMS) and the Society for Menstrual Cycle Research (SMCR). I assumed that without an institutional connection and outside funding, my dream would be just that. By the late summer of 1991, I was weary of expert analyses that tended to group women into large universal categories or anecdotal accounts without structure. I simply wanted to talk with them in a systematic way.

One night at the end of the summer of 1991, I could not sleep. It occurred to me I could do a two-year pilot study with 100 participants who would chart perhaps more than 2,000 menstrual cycles. At the same time, we would also follow what was happening with their multigenerational families. From this information, I might begin to see a range of experiences at menopause and learn if this was an effective way to approach it. I designed a flyer. At my regular Thursday lunch meeting for business and professional women, I stood to describe my plan for the project and invited interested volunteers. During my several years of reading, members of this group and other friends and colleagues had been approaching me to ask "What are you learning?" When I left the restaurant, I had a yellow pad with eight names and phone numbers. MAPS was launched.

Methods

Using the models from Bowen and Treloar, there were certain aspects of data gathering that were a given. There would be data books in which participants would record their cycles and add observations of interest to them. From enrollment, there would be a 3-or-4-generation family diagram charting each participant's relationship system, with particular emphasis on other women in the family and their reproductive histories as well as family patterns in reproduction.

While some other researchers were taking hormonal assays and recording lab values in addition to having women track their flows, I would stick to the areas I knew best utilizing methods accessible to the women themselves. I also committed to being myself from the first interview. I had a series of questions to ask about specific areas of information and planned to listen and document without intervening or giving advice. These decisions proved to be what made the project the most useful to the participants, particularly for those who stayed many years.

With quite a few, we simply had an annual check-in relationship. The women could count on me to follow their experiences with interest and without judgment. When relevant, I would also feel free to share examples from my experience and the range of experiences of other women, without pinpointing anyone in particular. I had learned from my clinical career that unless I was prepared to go home with people and live their lives for them, their decisions were strictly their own. I took the position validating each project participant as the expert on her own life, "the only person in the body." This approach, too, was valued by the women.

Participants

Between October 1991 and September 1992, 80 women enrolled in the research study. Nearing one year, I decided to close enrollment ahead of my original target number of 100 while continuing with those already participating. I could then concentrate on follow-up interviews.

Table 1.1 MAPS Demographic Data at Enrollment

Age Range (Number of women)	Partners (Percent of study group)	Childbirths (Percent of study group)	Parents (Percent of study group)	Highest Level of Education (Percent of study group)	Primary Occupation (Percent of study group)	Living situation (Percent of study group)
34–39 (22)	Married (75%)	0 (28%)	All living (47%)	High school (4%)	Health; mental health (24%)	With partner and their children (50%)
40–44 (31)	Cohabiting (6%)	1–2 (54%)	All deceased (11%)	Some college; Technical training (14%)	Government; Education (29%)	With partner only (30%)
45–49 (20)	Separated/ Divorced (13%)	3–4 (14%)	Mother living (27%)	Bachelors (41%)	Service; Clerical (18%)	With children only (9%)
50–54 (7)	Widowed (4%)	5 (4%)	Father living (14%)	Masters (35%)	Business (11%)	Living alone (11%)
	Single, never been married (4%)	Adoptions (4%)	Step-parent involved (1%)	EdS or PhD (6%)	Arts (9%) Homemaker (11%)	
TOTAL: 80	102% allows multiple roles	104% allows multiple roles	100%	100%	102% allows multiple roles	100%

Enrollment was by a convenience sample. Women came to the project through recruitment from professional and service groups, a newspaper ad, and a radio interview, but primarily from word-of-mouth. They presented varied menstrual and reproductive journeys, living situations at the time of enrollment, and family backgrounds, but were similar in the level of education (highly educated, a characteristic of both longitudinal studies and university communities) and ethnicity (white, including Hispanic). At the time of their enrollment, participants lived in the central United States of Kansas, Missouri, and Colorado. During the years of their participation, fifteen women moved from their enrollment cities (nine to another city in the same state, five out of state, and one out of the country) but continued with the study.

Through the 20 years of the study, from the first enrolled to the last data book received, participants reported changes in marital or relationship status; living situation; employment; residence; births, education, and launching of children; arrival of grandchildren; and illness and death of parents. Their evolving menstrual cycles were woven into the fabric of their families and everyday lives.

Process

The study began with two requirements for participation: (1) age between 35 and 55 and (2) still having menstrual flow. Due to a misunderstanding or insufficient information, two women arrived for their enrollment interviews at 34 years old; I enrolled them anyway. At enrollment, all participants agreed to commit two years to the project. The plan was for them to record their menstrual cycles in data books of generic calendars and participate in three personal interviews: enrollment, first-year follow-up, and second-year follow-up. Nearing the end of the first year and aware of the value of the incoming information, I asked each woman who returned for her first follow-up whether she would be willing to continue beyond the original two-year time frame. The great majority agreed to stay in the study, many commenting on the usefulness of the recording to them personally as well as their wish to contribute to knowledge for future generations of women.

Through the 20 years of the study, information was gathered in several ways. As long as women continued to have menstrual flows, they recorded that information in data books of calendars provided to them with the instruction to record flow ratings as well as the interval between flows. The data books also contained blank pages opposite each calendar for participants to add observations of their experience if they wished. For the blank pages, I simply told the participants, "If you're interested, I'm interested." Women took the opportunity to note as little or as much as they wished about their menstrual cycles and health in general, medical appointments or interventions,

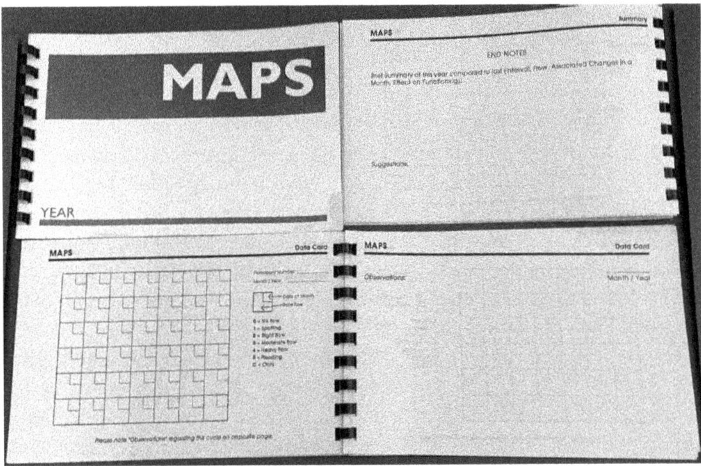

Figure 1.1 MAPS Data Book in 4 Views.jpg. Photograph by the author.

family and life events, and thoughts about living in a changing body. Many contributed personal reflections on aging.

The MAPS data book photo shows four parts to these spiral half-page books: The cover page gives the project name and year. Inside were blank calendar pages in which the women filled in dates and flow numbers according to the key given. Opposite to the calendar page was a blank page to record any observations about their experience that month and the final page in each year's book was a year-end summary.

For the first ten years of the study, I had personal contact with each continuing participant each year. Enrollment involved one-to-two-hour interviews, covering menstruation and reproduction, health history, and the construction of a multigenerational family diagram. Follow-up interviews typically lasted 20–60 minutes, reviewing the previous year's calendars and updating the family diagram, as well as noting health and life changes. For participants who had moved or lived out of town, data books were sometimes exchanged by mail, with interviews by telephone.

During the second ten years of the study, participating women who had documented a final menstrual period were given the option to continue through questionnaires tailored uniquely for them based on their personal histories and our previous follow-up interviews. This option fits with the fact that menopause is not a single moment in time, but a transition of many years, including before and after the final flow. Initially, these questionnaires were on paper, mailed to the women with a self-addressed stamped envelope; over time, some participants completed them electronically.

Differential Participation

Of the 80 women who enrolled, seven women never completed a data book, including two who did not attend a follow-up interview. Nevertheless, the baseline information they provided was useful and contributes to the total picture of the project. The information given at enrollment by all participants sets the stage for the prospective recording of facts that followed and is important in its own right.

Most participants recorded menstrual cycle facts in real time and gave at least one follow-up interview. Over half of the study population documented a final period during their time of participation. Those who left the study before recording their last cycles and/or before the end of data collection sometimes gave reasons for their decisions which were informative, shedding light on life in the middle years, the demands on women's time and energies, as well as their interests and beliefs. I appreciate the involvement and attention of each participant, regardless of how long each stayed with the project. Their contributions are an invaluable record in the continuing study of the menopause transition.

The Worth of Recording: Why We Do This Project

It's really pretty helpful to keep a record. I'm interested to continue.

It is interesting doing it. I really am pretty regular-surprised me.

I'm grateful I'm doing this. Really glad for the summary pages. Know I can come back and ask you.

It has been fun to participate in the study. I can come in and tell you things. You say, "Oh, yes" (that's what happens). I go, "Whew!" Fun to come in and update.

Sort of keeps me on top of things, too.

Been almost therapeutic – part of it is talking to you. I like that. It makes it more an important part of my life.

I want my film strip (alluding to the preparation we had for periods in junior high health classes).

No problem to continue, this is not very hard.

This has been really good, can go somewhere and be prepared.

Frankly, writing things down is not my cup of tea, but do think it's important. I don't mind.

I really appreciate that you are doing this. Has been really helpful. It has helped me have some perspective in the midst of all the funky stuff. Have the numbers right there, have to put them down. Sometimes I wonder where I am and can look back in the book for a perspective.

> I'm more regular than I thought I was in actually keeping track. I wouldn't want to be required to increase my data; I'm doing all I want to do. Making observations is what I'm interested in doing.
>
> I like keeping track. It is important for women to do.
>
> I will continue as long as it stays this simple. It will be valuable for me. Otherwise, I wouldn't keep track. It reduces some of the anxiety that I would have anyway. Having another woman to talk to about this, track record, communicate to doctor. Now that I'm keeping track I'm interested. Reduces some of the anxiety at this age. Feel like a pioneer-exciting-doctors don't know.
>
> Having someone care about my cycle.
>
> Strange to be writing this down when we've all been told not to talk about it. I think you should give back. This is a way to make things better for our daughters.
>
> I hope you keep up with this. I'm glad to continue. It forces me to do something that is important to do.

Longitudinal Studies of Midlife, Perimenopause and Menopause

What I didn't realize at the time MAPS began, other than the Treloar work, was multiple studies of perimenopause were also being launched, including The Melbourne Women's Midlife Health Project (MWMHP), The Seattle Midlife Women's Health Study (SMWHS), and The Study of Women's Health Across the Nation (SWAN). Many of the researchers who conducted these longitudinal studies of perimenopause made up the Staging Reproductive Aging Workshop (STRAW) in 2001 for the purpose of addressing the absence of a relevant staging system for female reproductive aging. STRAW was followed by ReSTAGE, a collaboration of those four large longitudinal studies to further explore and refine the stages identified by STRAW.

At the current time, STRAW+10 is an accepted model for staging reproductive aging. However, the journal *Women's Midlife Health* in its final issue (Harlow et al., 2023) offered an Editorial: "Women's midlife health: the unfinished health research agenda." The authors wrote, "One intriguing insight gained over the last quarter century, is the complex interplay among symptoms and physiologic risk factors, suggesting that more attentions to bi- and multi-directional relationships … is warranted." They added, "We need to remain vigilant to the unique and evolving stressors facing midlife women as they provide an important understanding of the social context for women's health." I suggest this is exactly where the methodology of MAPS and its offspring, the Multiple Continuum Assessment, can add an important dimension of fluidity and variant range alongside the mathematical studies of discrete variables.

However, if they are to be structured for the future, longitudinal studies such as those contributing to ReSTAGE and MAPS should have a place representing the complexity of life unfolding over time. There are many questions yet to be posed and answered, such as the one in a PubMed article from the National Center for Biotechnology Information (2020): "Is menopause still evolving? Evidence from a longitudinal study of multiethnic populations and its relevance to women's health," based on data from SWAN. The article concluded,

> The broad window of variation in age at menopause within the population and the absence of significant differences between populations, in combination with population variation in menopause symptoms, suggest that menopause is a relatively recently evolved and still evolving trait.

In the Commentary section of *Age and Aging* (2019:48:482–485), the authors opened, "Time is the best diagnostician." In an ever-shrinking, fast-paced world, individual women and their families, health care providers, and researchers often don't find the time or permission simply to let life unfold and observe what can be learned from it. The authors summarized "Longitudinal studies can provide data at many levels … trajectories of change in single or sequential cohorts … evidence of early predictors of later declines in health … and strengthen or refute evidence of causal relationships suggested by cross sectional data."

After 30 Years

Menopause is once again a hot topic as the next generation manages the passage, often in public view. Actress Gwyneth Paltrow at age 51 gives an interview on her "rollercoaster" perimenopause experience (Denham, 2023), while her mother, actress Blythe Danner, age 80, represents an osteoporosis medication on TV. In the ensuing decades from the burst of longitudinal studies of the 1990s, some things have changed, but the basics and need for useful information remain. Living in a time of dominant electronic communication, the opportunity abounds for both fruitful collaboration and rampant misinformation. Stress in general is shared collectively from person to person and country to country, increasing the pressure for quick, compact answers to complex topics. In this atmosphere, it has been recognized that more sound thinking about the menopause transition is needed.

The "first-ever" White House Initiative on Women's Health Research was announced (The White House Washington 2023) with the goal to "deliver concrete recommendations to advance women's health," and "engage scientific, private sector, and philanthropic communities." A number of sources are continuing to consider the need for solid research and to carry on the idea of longitudinal study. There has been attention paid to the general theme of stress in midlife, and interestingly, in "The challenges of midlife women" included in the previously cited Women's *Midlife Health* issue (2023) and based on a subset from the Seattle study, findings were that while "women found themselves searching for balance in the midst of multiple co-occurring stressors," they infrequently identified menopause per se as one of the stressors. Yet, multiple titles currently marketed seem to focus on the transition as a set of problems in need of fixing.

Reviewing recent literature, I've been pleased and refreshed to find thought-provoking and articulate treatments of perimenopausal and family systems research, multidisciplinary efforts in bio- and clinical medicine, neuroscience, philosophy of science, psychology, and anthropology. At the same time, I continue to see limitations in what seems to me to be the overfocus on symptoms, presented as slices and often reported with statistically dense data. While important in advancing medical knowledge, those examples do not communicate well with midlife women. Equally wanting is a popular literature that overdramatizes or, alternatively, mistakenly reassures, without allowing for individual differences and ranges of experience.

The appeal of the Multiple Continuum Assessment introduced in this book (Chapter 7) is that it is in tune with the movement of lived lives in midlife women through a natural process. The fact is family can be both burden and boon simultaneously, symptoms can arise, peak, and subside in short time frames and be all but forgotten not too longer afterward. What dominates and calls for intervention is within the context of many other variables in a woman's life. The continuity of personal annual interviews with the ever-changing family diagram as a backdrop in MAPS highlighted both challenge and resilience of the women, not only from woman to woman but also from one year to another in a given woman's life. Midlife women, their health care providers, and researchers aiming for insight into a fascinating phenomenon need better and more nimble ways to approach a moving target. The assessment template is flexible and can be utilized in multivariate situations, highlighting always nothing occurs in a vacuum.

The book is organized into three major parts. Part 1 introduces the founding of the project, its methodology, and the record by eras. Part 2 illustrates the value and possibilities of longitudinal work including the Multiple Continuum Assessment as a useful tool for considering the menopausal transition as an ongoing life process in context. Part 3 summarizes conclusions and recommendations for people in transition, health care providers, and researchers. It is hoped that this combination of research report, memoir, and commentary will challenge, serve, and facilitate increased understanding of the menopause transition now and in years to come.

References

Chan, S., Gomes, A., & Singh, R.S. (2020). Is menopause still evolving? Evidence from a longitudinal study of multiethnic populations and its relevance to women's health. *BMC Women's Health* 20(1):74. https://www. doi.org:10.1186/s12905-020-00932-B

Denham, J. (2023). Gwyneth Paltrow opens up about her "rollercoaster" perimenopause experience: The Goop founder, 51, got candid in a recent interview. https://www.redonline.co.uk/wellbeing/health/a45971237/gwyneth-paltro-menopause/

Harlow, S.D., Sievert, L.L., LaCroix, A.Z., Mishra, G.D., & Woods, N.F. (2023). Women's midlife health: the unfinished research agenda. *Women's Midlife Health* 9(1):7 https://doi.org/10.1186/s40695-023-00090-5

Harlow, S.D., Gass, M., Hall, J.E., Lobo, R., Maki, P., Rebar, R.W., Sherman, S., Sluss, P.M., & de Villieurs, T.J. for the STRAW+10 Collaborative Group. (2012). Executive summary of the Stages of Reproductive Aging Workshop +10: Addressing the unfinished agenda of staging reproductive aging. *Menopause* 19(4):387–395. North American Menopause Society. https://doi.org/10.1097/gme.0b013e31824d8f40

Keller, M.N., & Noone, R. J. Eds. (2020). *Handbook of Bowen Family Systems Theory and research methods: A systems model for family research.* New York and Abington: Routledge. ISBN: 978-1-138-47812-1.

Treloar, A.E., Boynton, R.E., Behn, B.G., & Brown, B.W. (1967). Variation of the human menstrual cycle through reproductive life. *International Journal of Fertility* 12(1 Pt 2):77–126.

The White House Washington. (2023). *Launch of White House initiative on women's health research.* https://www.whitehouse.gov/gpc/briefing-room/2023/11/17/launch-of-white-house-initiative-on-womens-health-research/

2 Early Years 1991–1996

When the women enrolled, I don't remember asking "what interests you to participate?" Maybe I was so eager to get on with collecting the facts of their lives it didn't occur to me. It's possible a few had already shared that when they volunteered, but I didn't record what they said. Nevertheless, by the time of the first-year follow-up interviews when I was polling whether people might be willing to stay beyond their original two-year commitment, I had my first glimpse what the project meant to them personally: the value of record-keeping, their experience being heard by another midlife woman, and their commitment to making a contribution to other women.

A participant who enrolled in her 30s answered the question "What were the pluses and minuses of recording for you?" "There were no minuses." She commented, "I am noticing changes in my body and what I am going through. I've always been real hit and miss; now I know to prepare in advance. It's a pleasure to know when things are going to happen." Another was less positive about recording but willing. She said, "Frankly, writing things down is not my cup of tea, but I do think it's important and I want to support you. I don't mind continuing."

I was very pleased that only two of the women declined to pursue participation after the first year. Both had busy lives. One indicated she kept up with the data book until summer but had gone back to school to major in engineering. On the one hand she thought it was good to have a record, but also wondered, "I'm not sure by observing it you don't change it." The other had never begun the data book, indicating she was "up to my ears in work" and "not going to be a very reliable subject."

By the conclusion of the study's fifth year, sixteen additional participants had withdrawn, including the only woman who died during the research project. She had been diagnosed with breast cancer following the birth of her second child two years prior to her enrollment in the study. After mastectomy, she chose not to continue with further treatment within conventional medicine and followed Christian Science, a great comfort to her. When her periods ceased she assumed it was menopause and I did not know what to think. She

DOI: 10.4324/9781003540830-3

had moved out of state with her family for her husband's job and we continued our updates by long-distance phone calls. When I received the sad news of her passing at age 42, I sent a letter to her bereaved husband with a note for their young sons for him to share when he thought it was appropriate. I wished to express my positive impressions of their mom and her keen interest to learn.

Other participants who withdrew from the project Years 2–5 represented different life experiences. There were those who had received answers to their questions about what was going on with them, including several who pursued hormone therapy, and were eager to get on with their lives. A participant who enrolled at age 43 said in her enrollment interview,

> It's my plan to do some kind of HRT, I'm interviewing physicians now. I have interviewed two, and have an appointment with a third. My husband asked me, "if you like the next doctor will you do this?' He's in there with me which is helpful."

In the first year of the study she began on sequential hormone therapy, switching to continuous combined in the second year. By the third year she had only one cycle to record and mailed her data book with a note: "Since I'm getting increasingly boring as far as my cycle goes, I'd rather not continue … I hope you've gotten useful information from me and others. I appreciate the work you're doing."

At the other end of the spectrum, another participant, who enrolled at age 47, discontinued the hormone therapy she was taking a few months after she joined the project. Having been hospitalized with panic attacks a couple of years earlier, she began seeing a psychiatrist for outpatient therapy and medication management. She said,

> If I was going through the change of life I really wanted to know. I'm willing to accept the changes going through my body rather than wondering what was going on. I waited and watched for a while to see if another period would start and then I forgot about it.

A few participants were focused on relationship and career changes which outweighed continuing with the project. A woman who had enrolled at age 39 had a variable cycle from the first years and was possibly in perimenopausal transition when she left the study in the fifth, saying, "My father is dying." Another who had enrolled at age 41 and was also in transition took a job out of the country in international nursing. Divorced with both sons in college, she said, "It was time for me to make a change."

And some, as the woman who withdrew in the first year, indicated they were not very good record-keepers.

Menstrual Cycles

Participants

At enrollment, each participant was asked four questions about her menstrual cycles: (1) Through your years of menstrual history, have you had a pattern which was recognizable to you? (2) Typically, do you have other changes in a month – physical, emotional, or relationship – which you associate with your menstrual cycle? (3) What effect, if any, does your menstrual cycle have on functioning-at home, work, school, or in your relationships? And (4) Have you experienced any recent changes in your menstrual cycles? As the women's ages at enrolled spanned 20 years, their answers to these questions provided a first look at possible stages to reproductive life as well as variables which could impact menstrual functioning. Women responded in terms of how their experiences had changed from their teenage years, to after first or second childbirths, and through times of stress. Two-thirds of the participants identified recent changes.

A woman who enrolled in her 40s described her history at enrollment:

I always had horrendously bad cramps. I prefer not to take drugs but I don't like to suffer either. Four months ago I took Advil for headache and had no cramps with my period. I have to take it soon enough or I will really feel sick-bowel changes, hot and cold. Last period I took one Advil and breezed right through. I don't know if it's my time of life or the Advil. My period over the years has shortened. I have lighter flow and PMS-type things-more sensitive, more inclined to be emotional-feel more like crying. For about a week before, I feel edgy … Sometimes my breasts get sore and sometimes they don't. My stomach is rounder a few days before. The mucus changes through the cycle. I feel more horny around ovulation. When I have cramps the first day they interrupt my life.

Also in her 40s, another participant commented,

I haven't been regular since I went off the pill. It's really unpredictable. I'm sick of carrying around pads. I don't usually have much warning-not a crampy person. The moon probably affects me as much as my menstrual cycle. My cycle has never inhibited my day-to-day life. Since going off the pill, it's extremely light in the beginning and the end. In the middle, it's heavier and a different consistency. I had hormone-related sweating for two to three months after I went off the pill-it was constant for a while, then it stopped.

> **Signs and Symptoms: Hot Flashes and Headaches;
> Insomnia and Weight Shifts**
>
> The hot flashes drive me insane! I am spacier than ever, but since I've always been spacey, this is not new.
>
> Periods of insomnia, 3 a.m., waking. Get up, feed the dog, walk around, have a cup of tea.
>
> I actually eat less than I ever have since I was about six, but I look more and more like a dumpling! However, so do my friends of similar vintage. And the good news is I am experiencing the best emotional health of my entire life, so it bothers me less.
>
> More abdominal midriff fat, "girthy" as my mother would say. I find willpower is not what it used to be although I hate tight waistbands.
>
> The hot flashes are mild and mostly amusing. They seem to be so normal as to be almost unnoticed as they have been part of my life for quite a while now. I find myself soggy, say 'Oh, yes, that was a hot flash.'
>
> Got rid of my osteopenia diagnosis. Exercise now is weight bearing as well as aerobic. Calcium, maybe one drink a week, used to be daily. Good things in terms of diet, health. St. John's Wort. Doing a lot more meditation stuff. Work out 5 days a week. Nice combination of things now, more up days than I've had in a long time.
>
> Still having periods and have also been getting migraines. They seem to come right at the day before or the day I start. Unpleasant surprise. Just wrote out a list of pain relievers. Have never taken them, need to experiment to get through that day or two. Can sleep it off. Need to be really, really quiet, no light, no movement. Hard to do when boys are there.
>
> When having hot flashes all day, pretty much was having a lot at night. Literally break out in adrenalin rush in cheeks. Head gets hot, have to start pulling clothes off. Have learned to dress in layers. Drenched at basketball game in November. At night don't have to change bedding. Have to throw off covers. Wake up. Cover up when cool down.

Reading the first data books, I was excited by the richness of the information. I had included as part of the data books a key for recording in the calendars. Participants were asked to rate flow from "0" signifying "no flow," to "5" for "flooding," with "spotting," "slight flow," "moderate flow," and "heavy flow" the markers in between. There was also a "C" to signify clots, a typical observation noted in the literature of the transitional era. I was delighted to find in the completed data books many participants had added to the key, tailoring it to their own personal experiences.

Early in the data collection I recognized a year's worth of menstrual cycle information could be depicted on a single sheet of graph paper. With months of a year the vertical axis and dates of the month the horizontal, it was a simple and straightforward process to plot participant flow ratings, count intervals between periods, and summarize at the bottom of the page averages and ranges. Also at the bottom of the page I could include categories of experiences participants mentioned in their observation pages. I had the impression the data was "talking" to me as the numbers "walked" across the page.

Women with approximately 30-day intervals had virtually vertically straight line graphs for the year whereas the pages of women with longer intervals walked to the right and those with shorter intervals walked to the left. Lack of pattern meant exactly that. Unusually short or long intervals and flows stood out visually; so did flooding episodes, "run-on" periods, and persistent spotting. I learned to associate which of these pictures caused management issues for participants, as well as to note what women chose to do about them. There seemed to be a continuum from women seeking medical help to those deciding to "live with it." Often what could be tolerated was based not so much in the menstrual cycle changes as in signs and symptoms categories such as "terrible sleep," hot flashes, night sweats, and headaches.

A participant who enrolled at age 47 described her journey at enrollment: "I was having really heavy periods with Tampax, pads and clotting, which gave way after a while to lighter and lighter. I stopped having periods for six months almost a year ago. Then I started again for five months, three of them consecutive. Then I stopped, had one, and haven't started now. When I'm not having periods I have real heavy hot flashes … I dread the feeling: all the muscles contract, then I fan and sweat. I dread when it will happen again. I've had frequent leg cramps, hot flashes definitely in my legs and my trunk. They squeeze and let go … The night sweats wake me up from a sound sleep. The feeling of being squeezed comes first, then I flip the covers off. During the summer I could have five to ten a night, now about once."

As women moved into the transitional era, some who were accustomed to having fairly regular cycles would note on the calendar the date they expected their period as well as the date it actually occurred. This was a meaningful, and for some participants a disorienting or disruptive, change. A participant who enrolled at age 45 said in her first interview,

> My typical cycle for the first 30 years was just like clockwork. The most variation would be 27–29 days. I was 40 when it changed; I went six weeks one time without; that's when I started thinking about menopause. Now I still mark on a 28-day cycle, but expect at 24.

During the first five years of the project, nine women documented their final menstrual period and of these, eight had hysterectomies (thus ending flow). One woman had an untreated menopause (without hormone therapy or any surgical procedures). Given the age range of participants it is remarkable in retrospect that over half of the women who had hysterectomies during the project had them in the first five years of the study. Some were quite young. A participant who enrolled at age 39 in 1991 said,

> I was on birth control pills from age 17 till 1983. I went off the pill with tubal ligation … Since the tubal, everything went well for two or three months, then a very heavy period. I thought I was hemorrhaging … Since then the periods have been heavier and totally irregular. I've had cramps for two years for which I take Anaprox. It's really hard to deal with.

Two years later she reported, I was taking Provera, then she took me off. Everything was fine, but slowly, heavier and heavier and closer together. About three months ago, the bottom dropped out … I am scheduled for a hysterectomy two weeks from today. I thought 'I am not going to deal with this'. My primary care doctor referred me to a gynecologist. I have tried drugs and I am not interested in being on long-term medication. My blood pressure is a factor. We talked some of a D & C, but I might just need something else later. Fibroids is what I have. It happened kind of fast."

Surgeries aside, eight women (10% of the whole study group from enrollment) had changes in cycles related to prescription hormones in the first five years of the study. Several tried hormones to manage difficult periods first and then had hysterectomies. I began to wonder whether I would ever see a "natural" menopause. One participant, who had enrolled at age 46 and had a history of heavy flows treated with D & C procedures, had her final D & C in Year 1 and hysterectomy in Year 2. While the most common reaction to hysterectomy for women with problem cycles was relief, this participant, who had not had children, commented "I felt like I owed God a big apology for not using the equipment He gave me."

Another woman, who had enrolled at age 48, was a teacher who reported in her initial interview she had begun the previous summer a sequential hormone therapy regimen to manage insomnia. In the first year of the study she arranged with her physician a plan of partial year hormone therapy which continued for the next several years. Then in Year 4 she had surgery for melanoma followed by a hysterectomy with oophorectomy for endometrial cancer in Year 5.

A participant who enrolled at age 38 had not yet experienced interval changes with her cycles but had a clotting disorder. This led to a hysterectomy when she hemorrhaged in Year 4 of the project. Another who had enrolled at the even younger age of 35 was prescribed hormone therapy for heavy periods in the second year of the study, and a D & C with hysteroscopy followed by a hysterectomy (for which she advocated) in Year 4. She reported findings of benign growths in her uterus. Findings on hysterectomy for other participants included endometriosis, adhesions, and fibroid tumors.

At the opposite end of the reproductive spectrum, two participants who had enrolled in their 30s documented their first full-term pregnancies during the first five years of the research. Two other women terminated unplanned pregnancies.

Researcher

During the first phase of the project while the women recorded flows and we exchanged completed data book for blank ones each year, I was getting grounded in the research field, in both menstrual cycle and family systems subject areas. Between the fall of 1991 and summer of 1997 I presented a number of papers based on information from the study at family systems meetings in Kansas City, Chicago, and Santa Rosa, CA. Topics ranged from the design and intent of the research project to first data collected, including patterns of reproductive behavior observed in the multigenerational family units.

In the same time frame I also attended the biannual meetings of the Society for Menstrual Cycle Research (SMCR) as well as several annual North American Menopause Society (NAMS) conferences, until the latter simply became too expensive and was not as central to me professionally. I found at the SMCR a multidisciplinary group which was welcoming, supportive, and largely female. My experience with NAMS was not as rewarding and I was reactive to it. The mostly male physician-dominated group seemed not particularly inviting to adjunct professions. I was also put off by the marked pharmaceutical presence at the conferences which was in turn reflected in many of the presentations. On one occasion, the papers from a group of anthropologists and sociologists presenting cultural comparisons on experiences of midlife women received a cool reception from the line of male physicians exiting the room as the speakers (all female) began. I did appreciate the words of one researcher advising his clinical colleagues "every woman is an 'n of 1'" but was baffled by the summary of another presenting his data on the use of HRT for women with risk factors as a "tremendous gain." I questioned how the population data could be applied to a single person. As a social worker and therapist, I wondered, "Does she want to live a few more months? What will be her quality of life? Who is in her support system? Does she have financial resources?" In those situations I felt similarly as I had reviewing the literature, that the "gulf" between professional frames of reference could be wide with midlife women falling in between. I admired female colleagues I knew from SMCR who had an important impact in NAMS and know my own sensitivity as an "outsider" prevented establishing good working relationships within that organization at that time.

In 1993 I presented a paper "Menstrual Pattern Change through the Human Life Cycle" (based on baseline and first-year data from the research project) at both the Midwest Symposium on Family Systems Theory and Therapy in

Chicago in May and the SMCR meeting in Boston, MA in June. It was well received by both groups. I was taken with how much the information spoke to midlife women attending, including other presenters. It felt like more of a risk with the menstrual cycle research group where I was a novice member than the family systems group where I was known and with which I was more familiar. The positive response to this paper gave me hope I could have a valid place and potential colleagues at SMCR, too.

My first paper in Chicago at the Midwest Symposium of Bowen Family Systems Theory and Therapy in May 1990 connected the beginning of my own research career with my father's. Appropriately enough, it was titled, "Reviewing Literature on Menopause: What is Science?" and was held at the Chicago Academy of Science where my dad had worked while I was in elementary school. Staying at a hotel walking distance from the Academy, the day before the meeting began I went over to acclimate myself to the building. Coming in at street level, I was a little disappointed not to connect to the place I remembered often having visited as a child. But going downstairs, the smell took me back immediately to my dad's lab! While he was at the Academy he had worked entirely as a research scientist before returning to academia in the move to Kansas. I asked the museum staff whether anyone happened to remember him. He had left in 1958 and died in 1979.

Fortunately, a young man generously dug deep into the files, giving me literally a treasure trove of my father's correspondence. The earliest letter in the file inquiring about a possible position was written when I was three years old and typed (I assume by my mother) with the all cap font of their old manual typewriter. The return address belonged to my paternal grandparents with whom we were living during the job search. Diving into this letter and those from the years that followed allowed me a heretofore unseen picture of my dad: young, enthusiastic, and eager to get to work after receiving his PhD. I was grateful to replace my working memories of his final years of illness with this healthy and extremely motivated person.

In the early years of the study, while I was building professional relation-ships and learning the many ways in which research could be conducted, I was simultaneously experiencing menstrual cycle changes similar to those recorded by participants in the study. I was in the same age group as the great-est number of women at enrollment, and while not an official participant, I continued to log my own data. Reviewing it now, I see in these years no outstanding variation in the interval, but flow changes that were shared by a number of the participants. Having the opportunity to follow these women eased my own reaction to uncomfortable aspects (spotting, heavy flows with clots). I realized "Nothing is happening to me that I haven't heard described by someone else."

I was also gaining glimpses of other changes that might lay ahead. There was a camaraderie in the shared experiences. Listening to a professional woman with very heavy flows describe the day she had to send her assistant to her home for a change of clothes prior to an important meeting, I remembered being in Santa Rosa in a white jumpsuit ready to present and questioning my choice. While I was spending untold dollars on disposable paper products I listened to a participant's memory of her mother's menopause as "the boxes of Kotex disappeared-we never talked about it."

General Health

Participants

At enrollment each participant was asked for diagnoses and treatments of any medical conditions, as well as medications and over-the-counter drugs or supplements taken, and history of hospitalizations, surgeries, or accidents. In addition, they were asked about substance use including alcohol, drugs, nicotine, and caffeine. At follow-up each year the women reported any changes in those categories from the previous year. A summary of their accounts reads more like an account of life in a certain geographic area at a specific time than a portrait of the particular lives of individual women and their families. This was especially true with regard to supplements taken and medications prescribed which reflected the influence of popular trends, both "expert" and informal, on women's choices and decisions. What I was reading on the covers of popular magazines and in professional journals came in the door with the women and their data books.

The participants had birth years ranging from 1936 to 1957 when they enrolled. At that time, the most common medical experiences mentioned besides usual viral illnesses and allergies were accidents, particularly in vehicles, and broken bones. Childhood tonsillectomy was the most frequently reported type of surgery, especially for women 40 and older. The diagnosis of thyroid conditions was more often noted by those 45 and older. I wondered about a possible connection with the hormonal changes of menopause particularly as the study continued and new thyroid problems were reported. Arthritis and joint problems also occurred with increasing frequency in the older age groups.

During the first five years of the project, eight participants had surgeries, including a couple of women with multiple procedures. These ranged from rotator cuff and gallbladder surgeries to tonsillectomy, breast reduction, and a lithotripsy procedure for kidney stones. One woman had surgery for melanoma in Year 4 of the study followed by the previously described hysterectomy with oophorectomy for endometrial cancer in Year 5. Two participants were diagnosed hypothyroid in the first years of the study. Three sought help for what they considered to be problem drinking. Documenting substance use reflected participant focus more than use estimates. Some women focused on caffeine, some on alcohol, some on nicotine, and a few on marijuana. In each instance, the reports were given in terms of "increase" or "decrease." No one thought they should have a goal of increased use of any of these substances while many mentioned efforts to decrease or discontinue and sometimes went up and down from year to year. Although I didn't ask specifically about diet and exercise, nearly half the women in the early years included them when responding to health questions. There was a general concern and monitoring of weight change, particularly its distribution, with the tendency to carry weight around the middle more than ever before. With respect to aging changes noted in their bodies, one participant in Year 4 was the first, but would not be the last, to mention skin wrinkles and said she was also aware of growing chin hairs.

Researcher

During the first years of the project, I did not have new medical diagnoses or treatment but learned more about what the previously identified asthma would require for management. The winter of 1996, which was stressful for other reasons, created conditions for the worst respiratory symptoms I had ever had. I learned wearing a ski mask for my walks in the sharp, cold air was exactly the wrong thing to do. I remember the dismissal I felt when a nurse (over the phone) told me, "You don't sound airless," countered by the ease I felt going to a conference in a hotel with a warm and humid pool area. As I learned what triggered symptoms and what helped, I adapted clothing and gear to be able to continue with year-round exercise in all the Kansas seasons. Delivering my first papers at conferences, I also became aware that anxiety could take my breath away. I learned using an inhaler before I was about to go on was as helpful for public speaking as for walking.

Fundamental to mental, physical, and spiritual health, I began a practice of daily meditation in 1993 at a time both my husband and daughter were out of town and I had the quiet house to myself. My mother had discovered Jon Kabat-Zinn while watching Bill Moyers' program Healing and the Mind (1995). She ordered Kabat-Zinn's first book *Full Catastrophe Living* (2013) and we practiced together at her house with the accompanying audiotapes. I ordered the book with tapes, too. Thus began the custom I continue to this day. When busy family life resumed, I put a sign on my study door, "Mommy Nomi is meditating," which was immediately respected by my family. Over time this daily habit, first a useful way to manage stress, became a way of life.

Family Relationships

At enrollment, I constructed with each participant her own 3-to-4 generation family diagram, according to the principles of Bowen Theory and along the lines recommended by Victoria Harrison (2018). For the women in the study, a central horizontal line placed them with their significant partners and spouses. The vertical lines included children in the next generation and parents and grandparents in the previous. Siblings of the participants as well as their aunts and uncles also were included. Bowen Theory emphasizes when building family diagrams the task is to focus on facts of the family rather than interesting stories or anecdotes. You may hear those along the way and some were recorded in my interview notes, but not on the diagram itself. It is also important to maintain awareness this is one family member's perspective which others might recall differently. In my own family I was at first surprised when visiting cemeteries or gathering birth and death certificates, that information I noted talking with other relatives differed from the "official records."

Family diagrams can include dates of births, deaths, marriages, divorces, educational level, degrees, and certificates, jobs, and geographic location to the extent any and all are known. It was my aim in this study to be as comprehensive as possible, creating for the participants who stayed the full 20 years a quite full 18" × 24" newsprint page! Given the research focus, I also asked participants specifically about the reproductive histories of the women in their families. Menarche age for female relatives was seldom known or even guessed at, and the participant's own, given retrospectively, could be reported as a school grade rather than an age or date. In turn, mother's menopause often was recalled as an anecdote or story rather than an age or date, with the exception of hysterectomy. Colorful recollections were part of my written notes, but not on the diagram.

As the family diagrams grew, many participants were motivated to learn more and would bring to our yearly updates additional information as it was learned over the years to come. Sisters in regular contact often shared about health issues, including aging and menopause. They were not, however, necessarily having the same experience. Those journeys within families as well as from one participant to another gave me another lens into variation.

At enrollment, nine of the 80 participants were living alone, four who had never married and five previously married. Half of the enrolling participants were living with their partners and children, most with children from that relationship, but some from a previous relationship, or both, in a blended family. Over a quarter of the women were living with a partner but no children while seven participants were living with their children but no partner. By the end of Year 5 nine women had separated from the partners they had been with at enrollment while one participant had begun and ended a cohabiting relationship during that time.

In the first years of the project three women who had previously divorced married their long-term partners. In Year 4 a participant who enrolled at age 48 said, "My significant other and I got married after 20 years. No one knew but my [adult] daughter which took lots of planning. It's a change but not really a change which is what we wanted." In the first year of the project another woman who had enrolled at age 43 married the man with whom she'd had a non-cohabiting relationship for 9 years. Diagnosed with a heart problem in his 20s he was hospitalized with arrhythmia twice in the first year of the project and sadly, died suddenly in Year 4 at the age of 49. A participant who had enrolled at age 46, married the man with whom she had been living for nearly 10 years in the fifth year of the study, which fit with an equally significant decision to leave her job of 19 years and pursue a new career. Also in Year 5, another participant who enrolled at age 36 and been previously divorced, married a man she had known 10 years but been seriously involved with for five months.

Those who had separated from partners identified different reasons. A participant who enrolled at age 40 said in the fifth year of the study,

> My husband and I just separated. It was a hard decision to get to and I have moments of thinking, "'What have I done?" He's very shocked … Everything is topsy-turvy in the family. Their view is how can I do this to them? But for the first time in my life I'm not accountable to someone; I was married more years than not. Turning 45 was a part of the decision as I've been re-examining my life.

Participants whose marriages continued sometimes referenced the effects of spousal job changes, health and stress levels on their relationship and the women's lives. A participant who enrolled at age 42 said at her third-year follow-up interview:

> This has been emotionally the hardest year of my life. I don't think it's my change. I think it's my husband. He's having a really rough time. I feel pretty strong but it was a real tough year. It came to a head on New Year's Eve. I'd rather get down to real issues than deal with superficial gunk; I don't know what's going to happen next.

The following year she reported, "My husband is still traveling quite a bit. We developed a contract … regarding economic decisions … It's been going quite well, actually." A participant who had enrolled at age 50 said at first-year follow-up,

> My husband has been making noises about changing work. We moved on average every two years for thirty years. He is always willing to move and I never wanted to. If he changes jobs we will stay in the region. I took my stand over a previous job change.

Fifty-six of the 80 participants at enrollment had given birth and two had adopted children. Nine had adult children who were out of the home, while thirteen women were actively "launching" children who were college freshman or high school seniors. Eight women had a mix of young children at home plus adult children, but the majority of the participants with children had offspring who were all under the age of 18.

During the first five years of the project the participants reported milestone events for children and stepchildren, including moving from one level of education to another, in and out (and sometimes back into) the family home, to college dorms and apartments, and in and out of relationships. They also noted medical diagnoses and treatments for their children. Four women recorded the marriages of their children, and three participants recorded their children's divorces or splits from significant others. Three women noted the births of grandchildren, while at the other end of the age spectrum, eleven participants recorded the first menstrual cycles of their daughters. Two women who documented full-term pregnancies during the project gave birth for the first time.

Four couples sought marital counseling in the first five years of the study and remained together through the documented end of the wife's participation in the project. Often, anxiety about children played a part in seeking help. A participant who enrolled at age 40 said in the first year of the study:

> The marriage is having some problems, we had a blow-up this morning. My husband has some things he wants to work out. I did schedule an hour with a counselor. There is enough stress in my life I can't pick up the slack like I used to. Our daughter moving out adds to the stress.

The effect of children leaving home could have both positive and negative effects on a marriage. A woman who enrolled at age 42 commented in Year 4, "It's been an interesting year; I'm happier in my marriage than I have ever been – I don't know what that has to do with getting the last kid out of the house … My husband and I have mellowed out." Another participant who enrolled at age 48 did not seek counseling with her husband until the focus was an estrangement from their adult son. She commented in Year 4, "My husband and I found out our relationship was harder to work with without our son – it's taking work." Finally, a woman who enrolled at age 49 and was married with four children said in her first-year follow-up interview,

> I've come to realize I need to try to center more on the relationship. I was raised to focus on caretaking. We have our granddaughter a lot. We've been able to keep the relationship better for both of us and make things better for her, too. I think the child needs to be considered.

Balancing the needs of oneself with the needs of others was to become key over the years in decisions managing the challenges of perimenopause and other aspects of midlife. This not only included relationships with the primary partner, children and grandchildren, but also with aging parents.

At enrollment, nine of the participants had already experienced the deaths of both parents. During the first five years, 13 women went through the deaths of a parent, sometimes the last living one, and a whopping 53 participants reported illness, including medical diagnosis and treatment, for their parents. A number of women mentioned cognitive decline in the older generation. A participant who had enrolled at age 47 commented in Year 3 her mother was "slowly going downhill. She has fallen once, takes walks, and reads the same thing over and over. I don't think she comprehends."

A clear sea change was occurring in the multigenerational unit. While some participants had parents who were alive and sufficiently active even to be of help with young grandchildren, it was increasingly the case that situations became reversed. The participant and her children could be called into caregiving roles with the eldest generation. Sometimes this involved the role of participants following a parent's hospitalization. In Year 5, a woman who had enrolled at age 42 reported her parents had been in her home while her mother recuperated from a stress fracture. She observed,

> We children are now more aware what mother is going through with father. They are now back home with lots of home health people coming in and sometimes she uses nursing home care for him … She would be better if Dad were not around; if he doesn't see her he'll think she's hurt and call 911. He has realized he is very dependent on her and she's not got a good attitude about it which my brother does not understand. I see it more after having them here.

With regard to her own health for the year, this participant commented, "Other than the two months of diarrhea I had when my parents were here which was very much stress-related, I'm fine."

Two of the women invited their widowed mothers to live in their homes, providing increasing support of different types in the waning years of their lives. One participant who had enrolled at age 38 and was the only child of her mother's second marriage described the situation in Year 4:

> Mother had cataract surgeries and struggled with depression a lot of the year, making the change from a very full life to wondering, "What am I here for?" It is hard for her when our family goes bicycling on Sunday afternoons and she is left on her own.

Two years earlier, the participant had commented about the extended family coming to her home for Thanksgiving. "They came because Mom is here, they didn't do that before she lived here. I put them on notice."

The illness and deaths of parents and parents-in-laws created a ripple effect not only for the participants, their partners, and their children, but also involved decision-making and role shifts with the participants' siblings.

Sometimes this became acrimonious. Two participants were party to lawsuits in their families of origin about questions of inheritance. Permanent rifts could develop. Sometimes siblings simply had different reactions to situations such as a parent's remarriage. A participant who enrolled at age 40 commented in Year 4,

> My [older] sister walks around like she has the whole world on her shoulders. After our mother died, things changed in the chemistry between us. I like my dad's wife; she is independent and good for my dad … My sister from a kid was always taking charge, now she's still taking charge as an adult; she's had blow-ups with Dad's wife.

Family diagram information was a key tool in assessing the degree of connectivity between family members, including geographic distance and knowledge about what was occurring with others. Many women with sisters made an effort to stay informed as to their experiences with midlife aging. In some families the sisters became resources to each other, sharing ideas and suggestions for managing symptoms. One participant who had enrolled at age 37 and came from a family of five girls began the habit of updating with each of her sisters before her annual MAPS follow-up interview.

Women whose mothers had already died or were cognitively incapacitated seemed aware of a void for potentially valuable information. A participant whose mother had died prior to her enrollment at age 43 reported in Year 2 she had talked with her paternal grandmother and her older sister. Her grandmother, then age 98, said she didn't know when she started her periods: "Oh, honey, that was so long ago." She didn't know what menopause was by that term. The participant's sister said she could bring on hot flashes "just by thinking about them," but her doctor had told her it could be several years before she would begin a hormone regimen if she opted for medication. The family diagram of this participant who updated for 19 years is replete with facts through time for her five siblings and their families as well as aunts, uncles, and cousins on both maternal and paternal lines, plus her own children and their children who arrived in later years of the study, and her husband's parents and younger sister. Her father had died in his 40s and her mother at 60, each with different cancers, but her family connections remained vibrant and alive.

Researcher

Like the greatest percentage of women in the study, I was living with both my husband and our school-age daughter when the project began. She was then 10 and hadn't yet had her first period. Although she and I attended a "Growing Up Female" class at her school sponsored by the local health department, she heard much more at home about menopause than menarche because of the study. Still, when her first menses arrived, she met me as I pulled into the garage after work, saying, "My red-headed cousin came to call today," using the old-time phrase we had learned in class. She was prepared.

On the other end of the age spectrum my mom turned 68 as the study began and in the previous summer had been diagnosed with endometrial cancer. I questioned whether the estrogen cream she had been prescribed for vaginal dryness might have contributed but did not receive medical confirmation. The same as her mother and three older sisters, she then had a hysterectomy with oophorectomy. I went with Mom to see a radiologist in Topeka about possible follow-up treatment. While their cancers were different my mother had lived through the effect of radiation on my father and did not think the statistical advantage the doctor quoted to her justified interfering with her independence and usual life activities. The OB-GYN who had performed her surgery supported her decision not to pursue radiation at that time and her subsequent long life (27 years cancer-free postsurgery) seemed to validate her choice.

Mom was always interested in the projects of her children, grandchildren, and eventually the great-grandchildren, and happy to see me begin the research study. We discussed what I was learning as MAPS continued. My husband and daughter accepted with equanimity the spillover onto the dining room table of files and books while I wrote papers. In the years I was first reviewing the literature, it was my husband who suggested how I could arrange my work schedule to free dedicated time for the research. It was a welcome oasis to have my own space for pure learning apart from regular daily life and obligations. My husband and daughter, with able help from his parents and my mom, all of whom lived in town, carried on while I traveled to meetings. The trips were not only professionally rewarding but also a refreshing change of scene which brought me a new appreciation for the comforts of home on my return.

Occasionally the meeting venues allowed for visits to extended family, too. In 1994 I attended the NAMS meeting in Cleveland and stayed with my cousin a year older than I. She and her family (our mothers were first cousins) had always included me in the summers we visited while my dad taught summer courses. She knew the role of Wulf Utian founding NAMS and regularly sent me articles from the local papers. Not only family members but also friends and colleagues aware of my interests also passed along information connected to the research, support I hadn't expected but certainly appreciated.

During the early years of data collection, my clinical practice was also going well. I arranged my schedule to accommodate both clients and research participants. I noted how much more relaxing doing the study was for me, simply partnering with participants in watching life unfold without the pressure to "fix" anything. Part of the clinical scene in that era was the advancement of managed care, creating tangles with referral sources and layers of burdensome, and often, it seemed to me, unnecessary requirements.

Life Situation: Career, Education, and Geographic Moves

Participants

At enrollment the family diagrams constructed with the participants included their levels of education or trainings, current employment, and geographic locations for themselves and their family members. Nearly a fifth had high school or some college, technical or professional education or training. The remaining 80 percent had college degrees, with nearly as many advanced degrees as Bachelors. A quarter of the participants were employed in the health and mental health fields, followed by education and business, and those who were homemakers. The project sample represented a number of different occupations, including in the arts, office management, government, and retired military.

The majority of participants at enrollment lived in northeast Kansas or northwestern Missouri with another woman in Colorado. Almost a third of the women lived nearby their extended families, while almost half of the participants lived not locally, but within 500 miles of their families of origin. The smallest percentage of the group lived more than 500 miles away, including half of that group living further than 1000 miles from family.

Distance became particularly important at times of aging and illness for parents, depending on the roles the women had in their families. Sometimes it meant leaving partners and children to care for parents, traveling back-and-forth while also working to maintain a presence at their jobs. By contrast, being readily available by geography sometimes meant being called frequently to serve as parental needs increased. This "on-call" experience was noted particularly if outside agencies and caretakers were involved. In some families, participants who had moved away from the traditional parental home found as they reached adulthood their aging parents joined them, sometimes a negotiated decision and sometimes not. The opposite situation occurred, too, when women who had lived near family found their parents retiring to faraway places. One participant, who enrolled at 36, and whose parents were divorced, lived in the same town as her dad but further from her mom. She was the oldest of three children of her parents' marriage. During the early years of the research project, her younger sister moved to the same town as the participant and their dad while the participant often maintained a health management role for him. Their youngest sibling (the only male) lived the furthest from all.

Reviewing the data from the five-year summaries now, I am struck by the number of employment changes for the women in the early years of the study. These included changing work locations, changing roles within the same organization, receiving promotions, changing schedules, quitting jobs, and beginning new ones. These shifts in turn had to be integrated within the life and finances of the family. A few women made multiple job changes in that five-year period. Several participants began new educational programs, while others completed degree work or certificate training. Each of those changes, too, could have repercussions for the whole family and their living situations. Over a quarter of the participants made geographic moves in the early years of the study, many as an outcome of relationship changes, including marital separation, and/or children leaving home. Some participants simply bought new homes in the same community, which had some continuity but also required adjustments.

Researcher

By the beginning of the research project I had completed my formal training in Bowen Theory, but continued to seek consultation from others experienced in the field. In an effort to secure possible funding for the study and receive what I assumed would be greater standing in the research community, I explored options for doctoral programs. I hoped I could maintain the research study already begun as my focus while obtaining a doctorate, but learned that was a naive assumption. I visited several campuses and communicated with other universities. In 1996–1997 I reached a turning point when I realized that what I was looking for in a degree program probably did not exist. It also didn't seem practical to become a commuter student taking on added financial burden while intending to contribute to our family income and maintain my clinical practice. I remember crying in a hotel room in St. Louis after an interview which confirmed my choice not to pursue another degree. At the same time the drumbeat of managed care grew louder and affected my private practice. Insurance company panels would expand and contract like accordions based solely on corporate bottom lines. I would be asked for my resume and malpractice insurance information, but no one questioned my approach to change.

Luckily for my own mental health, I sought personal consultations with two social workers whose work I respected a great deal. The first was a seasoned Bowen Theory colleague practicing in Chicago and conducting his own research project. The other was a professor at the University of Kansas School of Social Welfare for whom I had served as a research assistant during graduate school. Each listened to my plan for the research and continuing doubt how I would be regarded as a principal investigator with "just" an MSW. Then each in his own inimitable style validated the worth of the project and encouraged me that writing a book based on the interests with which I was most familiar would be entirely reasonable. Their message was: "You know these people the best; do it."

References

Harrison, V. (2018). *The family diagram & family research: An illustrated guide to tools for working with differentiation of self in one's family*. Houston, TX: Center for the Study of Natural Systems and the Family. www.csnsf.org ISBN: 978-1-5323-7664-1.

Kabat-Zinn, J. (2013). *Full Catastrophe living: Using the wisdom o your body and mind to face stress, pain, and illness*. Bantam, Rev Upd edition. ASIN: B00C4BA3UK.

Moyers, B. (1995). *Healing and the mind.* Main Street Books. ASIN: 0385476876. ISBN-13: 978-0385476874.

3   Middle Years 1997–2007

Introduction to the Middle Years

Whereas the first years of the research project were a true beginning, feeling our way as we went along, the middle years were a settling in, a solidifying of what the project was about and a foreshadowing of what it could become. Women who had self-selected into the study continued to select out, in increasingly predictable ways. Data gathering for the project ran like clockwork, or perhaps more aptly, "calendar work," as each year represented for the women 12 months in their data books. With some exceptions, our annual updates occurred about the same time each year. Participants shared with me not only structural changes they had made to their data books to fit their circumstances but also the habits they were developing with them, such as where they kept the books at their homes, how they handled recording when traveling, and the interest their spouses showed. Several women who had traditionally tracked their cycles maintained their usual routine through the year, then would transfer a year's information to the MAPS book for our updates. There were also a few participants who after hysterectomy without oophorectomy maintained data books for observations of their continued cycling.

I Divide the Middle Years in Two Sections: Part I – Years 6–10 (1997–2001) and Part II – Years 11–14 (2002–2007)

Middle Years I

During the second five years of the research project, nineteen participants withdrew from the study for a variety of reasons and at different menstrual stages. Three of the women who had documented their final menstrual periods (FMPs) by hysterectomy during the early years of the project and another who had documented hers while on hormone therapy left the project in Years 6–8. Additionally six participants I guessed to be in perimenopause transition withdrew prior to documenting an FMP. Four of the six had received hormone

DOI: 10.4324/9781003540830-4

therapy, while two women had continued with unmedicated menses. Those who had chosen hormone therapy based their decisions on symptoms they were having as well as family health factors.

A participant who had enrolled at age 47 reported at her Year 1 follow-up interview, "I went to a lecture by a doctor in which he recommended taking hormones if you were at risk for heart attack." Given her own diagnosis of mitral valve prolapse and fatal coronaries for her father at age 64 and an older brother at age 45, she opted for medicated cycles. Common in that era, this participant began first with a sequential regimen (Premphase) and later was switched to a continuous combined (Prempro). In Year 4, she had gallbladder surgery and was aware gallbladder disease was a risk factor with hormone therapy but remained comfortable with her decision. She reported the laparoscopic procedure was manageable with a single week of missed work.

Two participants who withdrew in the second five years had documented their FMPs without medical intervention, the first at age 43 and the second at age 54. The woman who had enrolled at age 42 did not use hormone therapy in perimenopause but had a menstrual history in which she took birth control pills from age 18, went off briefly with an IUD, and then returned to oral contraception until after her husband's vasectomy the year before her enrollment in the study. Her Year 1 data included a 21-day run-on period, and Year 2 had just four cycles, including what proved to be the final one, which was a brief five days of slight flow. After handing in her "blank book" (no flow for the year) in Year 3, she remained with the project for an additional nine years without significant health problems or using follow-up hormone therapy.

The woman who had enrolled at age 48 seemed transitional from Year 1 with an interval range of 16 to 40 days. By Year 3, the interval range had advanced from 14 to 102 days and she reported in Year 5 she had worn a pad "a couple of times" during the year which was "totally unnecessary. The last period I had was very circumspect." She also mentioned some spotting which she did not record. By Year 6 she described her final period: "I had to scrabble for some pads. It wasn't particularly overly long or short. We had gone camping and the period came out of the blue." Having decided the year prior she didn't see any reason to take hormones, she returned her blank data book in Year 7, opting to retire from the research project. She reported her doctor kept offering medical management for menopause which she kept refusing. She had clearly moved on with her life.

Three participants who withdrew in the second five years had enrolled in their 50s. Two of them had consistently used hormone therapy, one a synthetic regimen and the other a bioidentical. The third woman had experienced her last period six months prior to enrollment which couldn't be confirmed till the following year. She described her cycles had stayed the same till she was 54 when they "started getting more skimpy." Enrolling in June 1992, she retrospectively recalled a "normal" period June 1991, then "nothing again" until

12/14/1991 when she had had a "full-blown period with cramps, legs not with you. It lasted for about two days and I didn't feel like doing anything. I felt tired and weak. There's been no spotting or anything since."

Completing the first ten years of data collection, I saw a pattern whereby significant participant interest in the project matched maximum change in cycles and waned with no notable alteration on the one hand or by settling into a new life era with or without a documented final period. Three who withdrew in the second five years had enrolled at ages 35, 36, and 41, respectively and represent those who left before experiencing notable changes in their cycles during the project. They had, however, documented major life changes including relationship and career transitions.

Uncertainty and Change

Shockingly irregular-gets frustrating: 'Oh, again?' I feel like I have to walk around with a heavy pad, a light pad, and a change of underwear. No predictability.

I'm done trying to figure out when it's going to start. Only a few days when I'm not upon a period, having a period.

I guess there's a reason that twelve months is the gold standard. Please send me this year's booklet. After ten months, I got a period, can you believe it?

I really feel headed out, two periods back-to-back in February 'This is it.' Quite surprised in May.

It seems like one 8–12-hour period feels like I'm going to bleed to death, then it's over. Comes without warning a lot of times and with clots. Doctor says clots 'not normal.' I always hope I won't be out shopping.

No normal cycle, never know when to expect. The biggest thing – on several occasions hot for no reason.

Skipped a month, went two months. Went through two home pregnancy tests. Last period at three weeks.

After last year's visit, next period didn't come and didn't come. Only time I've missed a period. Got an over-the-counter pregnancy kit, lock door. Husband: 'Are you okay? What are you doing?' Since then, less regular than they were.

I've seen many changes in a short period this year but they're all *positive*.

I started fall semester wondering if there'd be health challenges and had my healthiest year in the last five. Life is good.

Still having periods. Lately every other week. No clue when.

Seemed like I had a period every time I turned around. For six months 2–4 days earlier. Then one that was longer-ready to get a pregnancy test. Do notice being weepy around period and at ovulation. Still really active physically.

Increasingly more like a 60-day interval. August or September truly the period from hell. Clotting, lasted a long time. General feeling of unwell. Chose not to make important decisions at that time.

Very important to ask, "What is this about?" Just an observation. Very curious about what brings on a hot flash. Only time has been uncomfortable was at a New Year's party. Wake up at night with puddle of water between breasts.

Periods seem to be reducing and reducing over time. Makes life easier. Sometimes more energized, too. That's kind of neat.

Menstrual Cycles and General Health

PARTICIPANTS

While results in the first five years of the project were weighted toward medically treated menopause, the second five years showed a more even division between those with hysterectomy and/or hormone treatment and those with an untreated close to menstrual life. During these years (1997–2001) four women had hysterectomies, all of whom remained active participants through the final years of the project. Two other participants documented their FMPs while on hormone therapy during Years 6–10 and stayed with the project past the 10-year mark. Seven women observed their FMPs without medical intervention, all of whom continued to participate past 10 years. It was a great benefit to our picture of the menopause transition to have participants not only document their final cycles, but also continue to describe their post menopause lives.

In the second five years of the project 21 women reported having taken hormone therapy of some type, including synthetic and bioidentical. Sometimes the move onto hormone replacement produced an immediately visible effect in their data books, more dramatically with the conventional medications. Participants recounted a more subtle experience with the bioidenticals, which I came to think of as perhaps a "softer landing" in the transitional phase. There was also a tendency to use them on a hit-or-miss basis "when I remember" rather than the conventional prescription medications for which they negotiated changes of regimens with their physicians. During this time three women had D & Cs, one who later had an endometrial ablation that led within six months to her final period. Two participants who had enrolled in their 30s terminated unplanned pregnancies and resumed cycling without significant change.

I continued to chart participant data collected along the same lines I had developed in the early years. My hypotheses about what I was seeing followed the idea of movement from one stage to another on the perimenopausal continuum. I noted changes in basic measures such as mean, mode, and range for flow patterns as well as the intervals between cycles over time. I also observed another trend. Simply by counting the number of medical diagnoses, treatments, and outcomes year by year for participants, I became aware a few women seemed to bear a disproportionate share of incidents, not only with regard to the project population, but also within their respective families.

Sometimes general health and menstrual events seemed intertwined and were hard to disentangle not only for me, but also for the participants and their medical providers. I knew from my initial literature review that reproductive aging could be treated as one topic within the larger journey from middle to older age. There was also a tendency for providers to put "menopause" in a treatment frame while addressing "just aging" as something common to all to be expected and tolerated. While I had the luxury of pondering the possibilities of mutually influencing variables, I was conscious of the stress involved for women seeking help interacting with multiple physicians from differing perspectives. Conflicting recommendations sometimes delayed their twin goals of symptom relief and return to normal life and functioning.

A participant who had enrolled at age 42 documented a number of serious conditions within a ten-year period, ranging from shoulder problems to vision impairment, shingles, and gallbladder surgery. Seemingly without a break from one challenge to another, the symptom which dominated the decade without resolution by the time of her last project update was migraine headache. Seeking recommendations from a number of sources, hormone therapy was at one point tried to ameliorate symptoms. At another time she was treated for hypertension at a "near stroke" level. The multiple challenges disturbed her normal life functioning to the extent she first went on medical leave from her professional position and ultimately retired.

Two other women who also had enrolled in their early 40s had significant medical diagnoses and treatment. Each had hysterectomy in the first years of the study which did not resolve their symptoms. Subsequent problems appeared sometimes within the area of reproductive functioning and at other times separate from it. Altogether they constituted a significant burden. Continuing to track family information as well as medical and life situation, I noted all three of the women were the oldest girls (although not necessarily firstborns) in their families of origin, well educated with responsible work histories, and often relied-on in their relationships with husbands, children, and siblings. When medical problems interfered with their functioning, it created consternation for them and their loved ones. Their family histories also reflected their mothers had suffered significantly more medical problems than their fathers and predeceased them, perhaps linking to a predisposition (vulnerability) to the pattern.

In the second five years of the study, a few participants had serious diagnoses (such as "hot spots on the brain") and procedures (such as lithotripsy for kidney stones), but seemed to recover without lingering effects or long-term disruption to daily functioning. Three participants noted anemias which appeared to be directly related to heavy menstrual bleeding and received iron. During this era a number of women had joint surgeries and were prescribed medications for osteopenia or osteoporosis, digestive ailments, hypertension, and stress-related anxiety and depression. Outpatient treatment for cysts of various types and bodily locations was common, sometimes several per person. Several women had accidents that required medical treatment, a couple of which involved alcohol abuse for which participants also sought help. Two women had face lifts and ten reported dental work, including braces, which were long-awaited and welcome.

RESEARCHER

Because of the skew toward hysterectomy at a younger age than so-called "natural" menopause plus the influence of hormone therapy on cycles, it would take me years to observe overall patterns in the transitional era. I continued consistently to complete graphs from each participant's annual data book and appreciated the wealth of material emerging. The two-pronged theoretical framework for the project, including family and life situation facts along with menstrual cycle changes, added a richness while also reflecting real life.

As I slowed down from the flurry of papers given during the early years of the study, I also benefited from a unique opportunity within the Bowen Theory community. Following a 1996 conference at Georgetown which invited researchers from the natural sciences to a dialog with family theorists, the idea was born to offer a Research Workshop "to train clinicians to conduct research on family process and related phenomena." I was happy to be invited to the first of these workshops in April 1997. The task was to present to our colleagues and the scientific consultants a description of our research projects accompanied by procedural questions for which we sought help. It was a freeing, informative, and inspiring experience to set aside the pressure of "expert" and obtain useful feedback.

For the second research workshop I attended in 1999 I introduced an idea I termed "multicontinuum analysis." Approaching the dynamic process at midlife this way allowed me to consider several dimensions of a given woman's experience at a single glance and was consistent with the concept of interlocking variables. I summarized the concept this way in a paper at the Midwest Symposium May 2000:

Data indicate that although the eventual outcome (cessation of menses) is the same for all the women, there is variation in the experience along the way in troublesomeness of symptoms, severity of interventions chosen to address symptoms, and the success of these interventions (as perceived by the person). These factors in turn interact with family variables, including the stability of the relationship network and the functional position of the person in that network.

The idea lived in me for the next 20 years awaiting the time I would have sufficient data from the MAPS sample as well as accumulated evidence from other studies to present a poster on Multicontinuum Analysis for the Society for Menstrual Cycle Research meeting in 2019. While I questioned in the intervening years whether I was really doing my job by not pushing the data to reveal more than it could earlier in the process, I was reassured by the fact Dr. Treloar had waited decades to publish findings from the MRH project, and Jane Goodall (1990) in the twentieth year of her Gombe research made observations that deeply challenged some of her previous assumptions. I was learning the reality of the patience required and opportunity presented by the process of longitudinal study.

Years 6–10 of the study brought progress in my perimenopause through to the documentation of my own FMP. In Year 6 I was still having an average (mean) interval of 27 days, but the range was from as few as 17 days in between periods to as many as 37. By the following year the interval range had expanded to 25–100 days with a mean of 38.4. In the final year the mean had jumped to 84 days, having had one 10-day period, followed by a five-day period 63 days later, and ending with 2 days of spotting 168 days after that. Plainly, there was no mode.

While I continued to learn to manage asthma, I had no new diagnoses or medications, although at different junctures during the research study my thyroid medication would be changed. Taking thyroid from early adolescence this was not new to me nor necessarily a function of menopausal changes. Sometimes the pharmaceutical industry played a part by discontinuing products and issuing others and at other times insurance requirements and coverage caused the shift.

Daily meditation practice continued to be foundational in my life, still on a solo basis. In 1996 I began walking for exercise which quickly became institutionalized as another daily resource. When I traveled for conferences, my routines came with me, helping me center in novel environments. I copied the women I saw in big cities wearing walking shoes between venues and switching to dress shoes for conferences. Along the way I began to pack a yoga travel mat and some of "my own food." Having eliminated dairy products from my diet in 1993 I became vegan for my 50th birthday in 1997. I regarded both as experiments to begin and found they "agreed with me" as my grandmother would have said. My menopause reading was an influencer in those decisions, particularly the introduction to the dietary habits of different cultures in conjunction with the presence or absence of midlife symptoms.

Family Relationships and Life Situation

PARTICIPANTS

During the second five years of the project, changes continued throughout the generations of participant families. In the primary relationship, five participants experienced breakups and another was briefly separated from her husband and then reconciled following counseling. Sadly, one woman was widowed suddenly when her husband of two years was killed in a light plane crash. The relationship breakups ranged from an off-and-on cohabiting relationship to a second divorce for a woman who had been married seven years. She and her husband had each been married and divorced previously and had children from their prior relationships. Two participants who divorced had been married for nearly 30 years and had adult children while another woman had been married seventeen years with a young child. In some instances, breakups coincided with other family stressors and milestones as well as a change in functioning for the spouse.

Project participants continued to mention stressors for their husbands, including job changes, health events, some of which were quite serious, and in one instance, a husband's retirement. One participant, who had enrolled at age 45 was significantly younger than her husband. She found herself providing support to both spouse and parents as they dealt with medical diagnoses and procedures. In Year 8 she reported,

> My husband and I just had a big discussion. He's retired and wants to travel. He is unhappy I'm not quitting my job to go with him. If something happened to him, I'm not old enough for social security which scares me to death … He's feeling like there's no time left for him … I never have a chance to just unwind and be by myself … When I retire I want to be here where I have my activities and friends. He is looking for an RV.

This couple was one of many who had to deal with different expectations at retirement, including both where and how to live. Often there would be peak points of challenge that had a way of working their way out with compromise and time.

Two women who had been previously divorced remarried during the second five years of the study and another began a new relationship. One participant, also divorced, who had maintained a non-cohabiting relationship with her partner for eight years, began sharing a residence as the children of their respective first marriages graduated high school and left home. In Year 2 of the study she had reported, "We have talked about living together but we don't parent at all alike. He goes outside when I discipline my son. We're just avoiding that whole thing." Eventually they moved in together and married two months before her son did.

While one of the participants who had given birth during the first five years of the project gave birth to her second son in the second five years, other women continued to launch their children. It was common for the participants' children to receive college degrees, but there were some who took a more circuitous route to adulthood. I admired the patient insight shown by women who could offer necessary (and ultimately, temporary) support, including their homes, to children when needed, while retaining the end goal of raising independent young adults. Again the value of the longitudinal study helped depict the full trajectory rather than an overfocus on short-term stuck places.

Given the age range of the participants, it made sense that as two participants documented the first menstrual cycles for their daughters in this era, seven others reported the births of grandchildren.

While some of the women were enjoying helping with their grandchildren, others were preoccupied with the illnesses and deaths of their parents. Sometimes those experiences overlapped. In addition to fourteen participants whose parents died during the second five years of the study, several women also noted the deaths of their in-laws and stepparents. It was not uncommon that cutoffs with stepparents followed the deaths of parents, particularly if the marriage had occurred later in life. Many women also documented the deaths of their aunts and uncles. The significance of each loss was embedded in the dynamic process of the particular family, requiring role adjustments to greater and lesser extents for the participants.

In Years 7–9 of the study, one participant, who had enrolled at age 40, expressed very well the situation of "the sandwich generation." The only child of her parents' marriage with an older half-brother from her mother's first marriage who was out of the picture in these years, she supported her parents through their end-stage illnesses while also offering backup to her son as he took steps to establish his own adult life. After her mother died, she brought her father to a facility nearer her home. Describing the toll on her own health, she said,

> I'm getting grayer by the week. It affects your whole outlook … I can't imagine what life will be like some day to have a weekend to myself. I feel like I'm the engine of the family-my son, my husband, my parents.

At the same time she continued to hold a responsible administrative position at her work. She commented, "I guess I kind of like it, too. I was trained for that. It's my role." The year her father's estate was settled she reported: "The burden is gone. You can't imagine my relief." Looking back on the caregiving years she commented, "It became an obsessive thing. I was real driven … It is a relief for me; domestic life is as calm as it's been in years and years and years." She and her husband were enjoying themselves and she described her son as "having a fine time-he's a really happy boy."

This participant was one of fourteen women in this era to report job changes and stress, including job advancement, scaling down work, and new positions. There was some creative combining of community contribution in both paid and volunteer capacities. One woman began doctoral work in her field and received the PhD four years later.

Thirteen participants reported geographic moves, including new home purchases in the same town, moves out of town, and sometimes several moves in the same area.

RESEARCHER

During the second five years of the study, my husband and I were also getting experiencing the life of the sandwich generation, as growth milestones for our daughter were accompanied by aging markers for our parents. In 1996, as our daughter finished junior high, my husband's parents and my mother were all able to attend the ceremonies at the end of the school year. By the time she graduated high school three years later, my mother could not even consider attending in the non-air-conditioned Allen Fieldhouse at KU, while my mother-in-law had to leave with a headache. In 1997 she had been hospitalized with postherpetic neuralgia as a result of shingles and never quite recovered her characteristic bounce as a vivacious "people-person." In 1999 she had a "mild" stroke in the summer following our daughter's high school graduation while her idiopathic high blood pressure remained resistant to treatment.

In February 2000, our daughter's freshman year at Grinnell College, my husband and I returned from a Sunday afternoon out to find a message on our answering machine from a doctor with Grinnell Regional Medical Center: "We have your daughter and she needs an appendectomy." After talking with both the physician and our daughter, we awaited news of successful surgery at our home, then drove 300 miles through the night to be with her. Once we knew the outcome, we contacted our parents. My in-laws were again "snow-birds," this time in Texas. I remember my mother-in-law saying, "It makes you want to see her." Several weeks later she experienced a major stroke, from which she never recovered speech. After several weeks of treatment in Texas, my father-in-law determined it would be better to bring her home. They returned to Lawrence but unfortunately, she never progressed sufficiently for home care, while he spent his days at the various facilities where she resided.

My own mother turned 75 in 1998, making her last solo trip to visit my sister and her family in northern California. Mom and I were also able to have a day of fun in Kansas City, the last one of those. At 80 she still would be managing in her own home, with home health care also involved. Through my daughter's high school years, I relied on her to also keep tabs on Grammy, and missed that when she left for college. Through the years the pattern shifted when our three generations went for walks. Originally my mom was the fastest walker and my young daughter the slowest. By the late 1990s, their positions had switched while I remained in the middle.

1996–1997 proved to be the low point of the private practice dip, and having resolved I was not going back to school in a formal way, I found the clinical work gaining ground again. This was helpful not only for feeling productive, but looking ahead to paying for our daughter's college tuition. When she left home, I changed my policy of accepting clients under 18. From the inception of my private practice in 1982, I had seen clients age 13 and above, including senior adults. It was a dicey issue for insurance companies when in accordance with my theoretical base, I insisted on seeing teenagers separately from their parents but still required parental involvement. The change to 18 and over in 1999 was a relief to me to not have the same argument with insurance companies (or families) over and over.

Middle Years II

The years 2002–2007 were significant in a number of ways. First, there was a new option in methods for the research project. A sizeable portion of participants who had documented FMPs and no longer required data books were interested to remain in the study to provide postmenopause information. Following completion of the tenth year, I made the decision that these women could be followed with personal questionnaires tailored specifically for them based on our typical follow-up interviews and consistent with the overall data gathering effort of the project. Continuing to track postmenopause reflected the understanding that the menopause transition is not one moment in time but a process over many years embedded in human lives and relationships.

Second, in the larger menopause field, the Women's Health Initiative (WHI) study in 2002 released results which had repercussions throughout the clinical and research worlds, and impacted the lives of the participants and recommendations they received from their medical providers.

Third, my own life in this time depicted the "sandwich generation" to a tee.

At Year 10, there were 22 participants who were eligible to continue with the project through personal questionnaires, having "graduated" from the need for a data book. Three were in the older age group at enrollment and had unusual recording experiences, including the woman who had her final period prior to enrollment, which could not be confirmed until her first-year follow-up interview. Another had been off and on various trials of bioidentical hormone regimens and was disappointed there was so little happening to log in her data book we discontinued it. The third woman began the study on sequential hormone replacement therapy (HRT) then switched to a continuous combined regimen in the first year, a common change recommended by prescribing physicians. During her second-year follow-up interview she described the final two months of the previous year, "That was the end of it."

Of the twenty-two, all but four participants elected to proceed with the questionnaire format. As the project went forward, some women when handing in their blank data books indicated interest to continue by questionnaire the following year, but when the time arrived for the next annual review, life or motivation had changed. Their involvement in the study effectively ended with the last in-person contact. Others noted the change from in-person interviews was an adjustment, not so much because completing the form was difficult, but that they missed our conversations. The majority adapted and many provided questionnaires until the project concluded.

When the study began in 1991, it was typical in medical offices for any midlife woman to have a discussion with her physician about what was then referred to as hormone replacement therapy (HRT), whether or not she was experiencing troublesome symptoms. There was a prevailing, although not universal, opinion that HRT would be helpful not only for managing the perimenopause but for the prevention of a number of medical conditions that might arise in the future. The participants in the study included in their updates hormone replacement regimens along with their other medications and supplements. Sometimes their decision-making process was included also. Since the project covered twenty years, it was not possible to compare dosages and treatment plans from one woman to another. It was even difficult to determine for individuals from one year to another. Instead I received a general impression through the years what the participants were typically being prescribed, as well as their adherence to and adjustment of regimens. Two broad divisions within the field were synthetic versus bioidentical hormones and short-term use for symptoms versus long-term use for prevention.

Ten years after MAPS enrollment the suspension of an important arm of the Women's Health Initiative (WHI) created consternation and challenge for thousands of women (Tanne 2004, Manson 2024). While I had been recording regimens and changes in them from year to year with each participant, the years immediately following the announcement were characterized by participants rethinking choices, new discussions, and sometimes even more change. A woman who had enrolled at age 45 and begun taking synthetic hormones in 1997 reported in her Year 10 follow-up interview: "The main reason I changed meds was all the studies that came out about hormones." In the years following there was further investigation which revealed methodological problems with the WHI, and the unusual way the suspension of that particular arm of the study had been announced to the public ahead of notifications to the scientific community and women's health care providers. (Bluming & Tavris, 2018). To date, the central divisions in hormone prescription remain, but the typical regimen has changed, both for dosage and length of use, perhaps an outcome of adjustments that were made in the early 2000s (NAMS Position Statement, 2022).

Menstrual Cycles and General Health

PARTICIPANTS

In the early years of the project twelve participants had documented the end to their flows, nine of them through hysterectomy. Two had untreated menstrual cycles, while the twelfth was the participant previously described whose menstruation potentially ceased with a presumed breast cancer metastasis. During 1997–2001 (Middle Years I), another twelve participants documented their final menstruations, three by hysterectomy, two with continuous use of hormone therapy, and seven with essentially untreated menstrual cycles although a couple women had used hormones briefly for symptoms not tied to the time of the last period.

In the third five years 2002–2007, eleven women withdrew from the project, all but four of whom were transitional at the time, but had not yet documented their FMP. Fifteen women did document final menses during this era, the greatest number in any five-year segment of the study. Middle Years II continued the trend toward untreated menopause. There were two participants with hysterectomies and another whose periods ceased nine months following an endometrial ablation. Whereas the average age for those having surgical menopause in the early years was 45 which increased in the middle years of the study, it remained lower than the average age for unmedicated menopause in all eras of the project.

Two participants documented their final flows in the Middle II era of the project due to cancer diagnoses, one with hysterectomy for endometrial cancer and the other following surgery and chemotherapy for breast cancer. Prior to their final periods, they each had provided at least ten years of menstrual cycle information.

The participant who eventually had hysterectomy had enrolled in the research project the month before her 37th birthday. Her first year in the study she had a miscarriage, followed by a D & C and an endometrial biopsy. She recorded a double-digit interval range with an average of 27. She had a tendency to extended flows including a number of days of spotting. In Year 2 she was pregnant and gave birth by C-section to her only child. Year 3 showed a return to her former pattern of spotting and a mode of 27. Years 4–7 included single digit interval ranges with typical means of 25.6–26.7 and flow averages of about 8 days. In Year 8 she had a run-on period of 32 days while preparing to sell her home in anticipation of a move to her hometown. She had divorced and her parents had each been diagnosed with serious illness. In Year 9 she had multiple months without flow while using oral contraception which had been prescribed to address "irregular periods." She later reported, "I went off the pill because I got feedback if I stayed on without flow I would have to have an endometrial biopsy."

Years 10 and 11 were fairly typical, but she had a run-on period in the last months of Year 12. In the aftermath she wrote:

> I'm very grateful you're doing the menopause study and I'm glad I've stuck with it over the years. Perhaps being a part of the study has helped me be more "aware." I had a recent month of 31 days of flow before having a D & C with endometrial biopsy. Endometrial cancer diagnosis-stage 1 … very early. I just took in that book three times and showed the docs, copied March and April flow when I thought things were really out of hand and got a response! Just one month of weird flow and I was able to be on it.

Following her hysterectomy with oophorectomy, she remained in the research project for three additional years, during which time she remarried after experiencing the deaths of both her parents.

The participant who eventually had surgery for breast cancer had enrolled at age 44. Her Year 1 showed a typical cycle, with a single digit interval range, average interval of 29 days with 4–5 days of menstrual flow. She documented no flooding, run-on periods, or extended days of spotting. Year 2 showed one 33-day interval, but the average remained 29. There were three months in that year in which she recorded "D" for a colored discharge, distinct from her notation of "1" for spotting. She continued with a stable average interval of 28–31 until Year 8. In the tenth month of the data book for that year she recorded a run-on period with flooding and 18 days of either discharge or flow. The following month she was prescribed Premphase hormone therapy which was switched to Prempro in Year 9. With the hormone treatment the interval became more variable than in previous years and was accompanied by lighter flows. In March 2001 she skipped her period altogether and recorded an interval range for Year 10 of 15–121 days with an average of 41. In November she had a D & C for "irregular periods" and a benign polyp was removed. Then in December her mammogram led to a needle biopsy. A double mastectomy with tram flap reconstruction was scheduled for the following month. After surgery her first chemotherapy treatment was in March, followed in April by her first period since December, then her second chemotherapy treatment and FMP in Year 10.

When she arrived for her Year 10 follow-up she announced, "Your paper's not big enough," referring to the multigenerational family diagram and reflecting the eventful year she had had, which included not only her own medical journey but the death of her father with an astrocytoma. The participant reported "Hospice was wonderful-he withered away to nothing in 22 days" and died in August. About her own experience with double mastectomy, she shared her thinking: "I am not going to go through this twice." As it turned out cancer was found in both breasts. She had stopped taking the hormone therapy in November when her gynecologist told her, "Your uterus is so thin, I don't see any reason for you to take it." Following her mastectomy her oncologist said, "We will shut you down with this chemo." She reported, "It upsets me something terrible just going in that office" and experienced headaches after treatments, "one of those sick headaches where you throw up. I have days I'm really tired; the first 5–6 days after chemo I'm really exhausted." The plan was for four rounds of chemotherapy followed by tamoxifen. "Losing my breast was no big deal but this chemo." She had praise for her surgeons and said, "My husband has been there the whole time. He has been wonderful. He didn't really want me to have the reconstruction, thought it would be too traumatic, but now says, 'I think you did the right thing.'" The participant did one more in-person interview, turning in her blank book in Year 11 saying, "It's great not having periods anymore." Eventually she discontinued the tamoxifen after experiencing side effects and continued to update with questionnaires through the final year of the research project.

Including the participant with hysterectomy for endometrial cancer in the first year of the study, for every woman diagnosed with cancer during the research project, the diagnosis coincided with multiple major life and family events. Happily each of them benefited from successful treatment and survived their illnesses throughout the time of their research project participation.

For the group at large, the majority of those participants documenting their FMPs in the third era of the study were able to do so without life-threatening illness or trauma. For example, the menstrual courses of three participants who also documented their final periods during Middle Years II reflected common elements of moving through the menopause transition relatively smoothly and without incident. Two of them had enrolled at age 38 and the other at age 40. All experienced their final menstrual cycles at the age of 52, and each contributed at least 14 consecutive years of information. One woman did not opt to continue by the questionnaire following her final data book interview, another contributed two questionnaire updates, and the third remained in the project till the end. All had untreated cycles without surgical procedures or hormone therapy of any type. None had debilitating symptoms which interfered with their functioning, and all worked steadily throughout, self-employed in their respective professions.

Each of those participants did observe family milestone events during this era. One woman and her husband divorced after their adult children left home ostensibly due to having differing goals for later life. They both began new relationships following the divorce. The participant's father, who had been widowed immediately prior to her enrollment in the project, remarried, and her own first grandchild was born. The eldest child of one of the other women received her first college degree and was headed for medical school. This participant had been diagnosed with anemia due to heavy periods and prescribed iron while continuing with her regular life and responsibilities. The third woman launched her youngest child, noted her husband had had a career change, and that her mother had died following a long illness. There was uproar in her family for a bit of time when her oldest son and his girlfriend had their first child, the participant's first grandchild. She needed to deal with reactivity in her marriage and with her father, which seemed to be settling down as she left the project.

The Year 1 data books for these three participants show single digit interval ranges with average intervals and modes ranging from 26 to 33. At Year 5 the modal range narrowed from 27 to 31 with a little more variation around the mean. In Year 10, one participant had an interval range of 18–120 days, another had 18–44 days, and the third had 24–52 days. Modes ranged from 26 to 29. None of the women were experiencing run-on periods, one described a little more spotting than the other two, and the third was typically having one day of flow per cycle she noted as a "5" for "flooding." They documented their final periods in consecutive years of the study, Years 13, 14, and 15.

In this five-year era, the most common medical diagnoses for participants were osteopenia or osteoporosis, elevated cholesterol, problem joints, diagnosis and treatment of cysts, and mental health issues such as anxiety and depression. Medications and supplements reported matched those diagnoses as well as including conditions such as digestive upset and low iron counts. It seemed to me by percentage, I was hearing about more falls resulting in more serious injury to them as well as vehicular accidents for the women as they aged.

RESEARCHER

2002 established that my final menstrual cycle had in fact occurred the previous year. Having experienced menarche at age 9 and completed my family, I was more than ready to be done with menstrual periods. I was aware of some hot flashes, but found nothing moving into postmenopause was troublesome in the way the years of heavy frequent flows in perimenopause had been. Even then, however, nothing had happened that required medical management. Being in contact with so many women on their own midlife journeys gave me perspective and patience with the changes I might not otherwise have had.

2002 was also the year of my final attendance at the Research Workshop at Georgetown. I presented to the group my plan for a methodology change in the study to follow the women continuing in the project post menopause. I received an encouraging comment regarding the concept for a personalized questionnaire, "I would much rather answer something that has to do with me," which helped solidify my decision.

Within this particular 5-year period, my experience presenting at a Society for Menstrual Cycle Research meeting in 2005 was not as positive. Partly, the difficulty was due to a new and quite specific physical problem. Surfacing to intolerable levels the first week of 2005 I was diagnosed after a number of weeks by a specialist with "noise-induced high-frequency hearing loss with recruitment." The hearing loss itself is not so unusual, and to some extent predicted considering my gender, age, exposure to loud music as a teenager, and having attended decibel-shattering indoor sporting events. The "with recruitment" aspect was the challenge that interfered with my work and life enjoyment, and required management. My understanding is "with recruitment," our bodies try to compensate for a damaged frequency by developing extra sensitivity in those surrounding it. I described my hearing as "amplified." I used specialized ear plugs and noise-canceling devices of one type or another to be able to function with as little pain as possible as all sound (except bird song) became noise, at times excruciating if the frequency hit directly on the damaged area.

While contending with the most acute phase of the hearing problem, I drove to Boulder, CO to give a paper at the SMCR biannual conference. Titled "Family Position, Personal Experience and Decision-Making at Menopause," I was excited to bring together my two areas of research interest. Looking at the confused faces of dear colleagues, I realized a brief paper was not going to do it. I had missed the mark attempting to bridge different vocabularies and varying perspectives. I knew the group wished to be supportive, but between the physical pain from exposure to a noisy situation, and the emotional sting of disconnection, I felt isolated and lonely during this meeting.

The best part of the trip was I had provided myself two days of respite at a small room in the mountains for quiet time ahead of the conference. When I came back to town, I found a book store on Pearl Street, one of my most grounding activities in any city. There I bought my first book by Thich Nhat Hanh (1999), never dreaming the significance his life and practice would have on my own. Heading home, I felt proud I had made the drive to Boulder by myself (a first), and resolved to do a better job the next opportunity to communicate family systems-based concepts to menstrual cycle research groups. Seemingly out of nowhere a song kept singing itself to me and I sang along all the way home: "There is ample time for all things."

This proved to be true for the hearing problem. When first diagnosed, my otolaryngologist (ENT) told me that 90% of those diagnosed with recruitment experience decreased intensity within two years, and in my case, it was, thankfully, 19 months. Sitting meditation one morning I realized my hearing was not quite as sensitive. Reporting that to my husband, we both cried. He was well aware the challenge it had been for me to continue to meet with clients and come home with raging headaches that sent me right to bed. It had affected our social life too. I had withdrawn from or adapted a number of my usual activities including lunches with my women friends. Restaurants could be intolerably noisy with overlapping conversations and the clanking of silverware. My husband and friends were solicitous to my need to put "my bad ear" to a wall, as well as which public venues to avoid altogether.

Family Relationships and Life Situation

PARTICIPANTS

In the third era of the study, participants continued to report family changes. In their primary relationships, two women divorced, one after seventeen years of marriage and the other after seven. Seven participants who had been previously divorced began new relationships; and three women remarried. One married her partner after cohabiting for eight years and another had a civil ceremony with her same-sex partner, with whom she had been in a relationship for five years. The women remaining in the study also continued to report important changes for their partners including work, health, and legal issues.

Many of the children of the participants received technical accreditation and/or educational degrees from Associates to Masters. Some adult children married, some divorced, and ten had children of their own. Many of the children made geographic moves, both to and away from the hometown and participants who lived near grandchildren often were involved in their care. Those who lived more distantly incorporated regular visits into their lives. Two participants reported their youngest or only children had graduated high school emptying the nest.

Eleven women experienced the deaths of their parents. For five of them it was their fathers, for six the deaths of their mothers. For seven participants this death represented their last living parent. I was familiar from clinical training that whatever one's age when the last parent dies, there is an identifiable experience of orphanhood, unique for each person in the context of her own family. I had known going into the research project that menopause was a process of years, and as we documented the physical changes we were simultaneously observing change over time in generational relationships.

Along with the serious illness or deaths of parents, participants were also reporting significant losses in their families of other relatives, including siblings, aunts, uncles, and in one instance, the sad suicide of a nephew, who had been the only member of his generation. Another woman reported the death of a nephew with brain tumor and melanoma at the age of 25 following the pattern of his father (her brother) who had died with a brain tumor at age 45, and his grandfather, their father, who died with a brain tumor at age 31. Listening to these histories I was witness to the remarkable resilience of families in the face of significant threats as well as the multiple ways there are to establish and maintain bonds.

None of the women participating during this era reported educational milestones for themselves; the focus in that area went increasingly to the achievements of children. Thirteen of the women moved, seven within their same town, five to cities in the same state, and one out of state.

RESEARCHER

Throughout 2002, my mother-in-law's health continued to fail until, after several false alarms, we received the call Christmas night she had died. Our daughter, who had been home from college for Thanksgiving when her grandmother was nearing her final hospitalization was home then too. During her winter break, she planned after New Year's to visit her fiancé. Having met as summer college staff at Ghost Ranch in New Mexico the summer of 2001 they had returned to their respective colleges and become engaged spring break of 2002. He had been with us the previous Thanksgiving and I could only think then how different his meeting my mother-in-law would have been prior to her stroke. My sister and her family were also visiting the week following Christmas and she kindly brought our mom to the service for my mother-in-law. My husband included a poem by our daughter about her grandma as part of his eulogy for her. One of our daughter's childhood friends who had known my in-laws well and enjoyed traveling with them, sang "Amazing Grace." With my daughter and sister both leaving town in early 2003 the weight of responsibility for my mom felt heavier than ever.

That year brought a number of significant changes. Our daughter graduated college in May and planned to marry in August. Her fiancé, two years older than she, had finished his Bachelor's degree and was already in Missoula, MT to establish residency toward his Masters. She joined him the summer of 2003, while planning their "distance wedding" at Ghost Ranch. Considering the conditions and her limitations, my mom stayed in Lawrence but my father-in-law and his new companion were able to attend, traveling with my husband's sister and her husband.

In the spring my father-in-law had begun to see a widow he and my mother-in-law had known when the couples were part of a social group who enjoyed dancing. His new relationship quickly became so important she attended our daughter's college graduation in May and her wedding in August. In the fall, my father-in-law sold his home in our hometown and moved 20 miles to the west to live with his new partner in her home. While they never married, they shared residences till the end of his life as she partnered him and helped to manage his mounting health challenges. Updating the family diagrams for the women in the study, I had been aware of vertical and horizontal growth and losses. This era I was seeing both on my own diagram as well.

In October 2003, my mother celebrated her 80th birthday for which my sister and I and our husbands invited a small group to her home for a little party. The guest list consisted of five long-time friends, and four caregivers who had become friends. The following summer my mother was hospitalized for only the fourth time in her long life (including two childbirths and the 1991 hysterectomy). Diagnosed with parvovirus she spent 12 days in the hospital, including stays on both the medical and rehabilitation floors. Her physician with whom I'd worked in a professional capacity was supportive with my "taking report" to pass on to my sister, the nurse. I underlined that Mom's goal was to return to her own home where she lived alone. She needed to be able to cope sufficiently with available outpatient resources on discharge. Mom did continue to "age in place," her preference, for another decade.

The Middle Years II era of the study culminated for me personally with another addition to our family, my first grandchild and my mother's namesake. My husband and I traveled to Missoula to be present for the birth in our new (to us) mini-motorhome with two little dogs we had adopted from the local Humane Society. Over the somewhat sketchy mountain airwaves, we took long-distance phone calls from my mother and his father wondering just when their first great grandchild would arrive. From the time it became clear how settled our daughter was becoming west of the Rockies, the appeal to be nearer occupied our minds.

The closest we came in this era was a trip to Flagstaff in 2006, seriously contemplating what a move might entail and the possibilities for life there. While I was quite disappointed at the time, it was lucky we opted not to go. Potential new colleagues shared they couldn't afford to buy their own homes given skyrocketing housing values, a foreshadowing of what would occur with the upside-down mortgage situation of 2008. We also learned the recreational opportunities we had envisioned were not quite the same in reality once there, and not as easily combined with work as we might have imagined.

Coming home, I realized I needed to approach Lawrence, my hometown, in the same way I approached new communities. Reading books by Thich Nhat Hanh I had received the consistent message that practicing meditation in a group was an important experience different than solo. I joined a local Lawrence sangha (mindfulness meditation community), broadening my horizons while also continuing daily meditation at home. I also began attending the meetings of the Douglas County Coalition on Aging, relevant for my professional interests, but also for my mom and me. When we had traveled to Flagstaff I had investigated options for a move for her, too, thinking it was unlikely she would want to remain in Lawrence without a daughter. A move to my sister's town had been tried in 1991 but was not a good fit for either of them. As it turned out, my husband and I did not move, and neither did Mom.

References

Bluming, A., & Tavris, C. (2018). *Estrogen matters: Why taking hormones in menopause can improve women's well-being and lengthen their lives-without raising the risk of breast cancer*. New York: Little, Brown Spark Hachette Book Group. ISBN-13: 978-0-316-48120-5.

Goodall, J. (1990). *Through a window: My thirty years with the chimpanzees of Gombe*. Boston, MA: Houghton Mifflin Company. ISBN-13: 978-0547336954.

Manson, J.E., Crandall, C.J., Rossouw, J.E., Chlebowski, R.T., Anderson, G.L., Stefanik, M.L., Aragaki, A.K., Cauley, J.A., Wells, G.L., LaCroix, A.Z., Thomson, C.A., Neuhouser, M.L., Van Horn, L., Kooperberg, C., Howard, B.V., Tinker, L.F., Wactawski-Wende, J., Shumaker, S.A., & Prentice, R.L. (2024). The Women's Health Initiative randomized trials and clinical practice a review. *JAMA*. https://doi.org/10.1001/jama.2024.6542

NAMS Position Statement (2022). The 2022 hormone therapy position statement of The North American Menopause Society. *Menopause: The Journal of the North American Menopause Society* 29(7):767–794. https://doi.org/10.1097/GME.0000000000002028

Nhat Hanh, T. (1999). *The miracle of mindfulness: An introduction to the practice of meditation*. Boston, MA: Beacon Press.

Tanne, J.H. (2004). Oestrogen arm of women's health initiative trial is stopped. *BMJ* 2004:328. https://doi.org/10.1136/bmj.328.7440.602

4   Final Years 2008–2012

The final years of the project brought not only great rewards in the number of participants who stayed till the end but also a breakthrough in analyzing their menstrual cycle data that would connect our results to those from major longitudinal studies the world over. It was also a significant time in my personal life on health, family, and career fronts.

Previously in this account, I have opened each 5-year section of the 20-year project with a summary of women who withdrew during that period, and the variety of situations and patterns of participation they represented. From the early years on, I understood each person had made an initial 2-year commitment to a "pilot project" which the overwhelming majority kept. The information each participant contributed for however long she stayed was valuable in this essentially exploratory study. With Year 10 and the addition of the new method, the summary included those who had documented their final menstrual periods (FMPs) but were willing to complete personalized questionnaires on annual follow-up. Now addressing the final years of the study, I concentrate on the participants who supplied continuing information over the greatest number of years, as well as the closing numbers for the project.

Thirty-two women remained with the project to begin the Final Years, including 22 who went the 20-year distance. The Final Years group included nine women who had enrolled at age 34–39, sixteen at ages 40–44, five at ages 45–49, and two from the oldest cohort in the study having enrolled when they were 50–55 years old.

Menstrual Cycles

Participants & Researcher

Having completed 20 years of data collection, it is possible to summarize the findings. Forty-nine of the original 80 women documented their FMPs while participating in the research project, including fourteen through hysterectomy and one nine months after an endometrial ablation. From the surgery group we learned those ending menstruation through hysterectomy did so on an average

DOI: 10.4324/9781003540830-5

at younger ages than those who did not. It took another decade to learn which data were significant on the road to menopause for those with medicated or unmedicated cycles and without surgical procedures.

The hysterectomy group contained two women diagnosed with endometrial cancer who had also had histories of hormone use. Another participant having hysterectomy had a bleeding disorder from which she hemorrhaged during a particularly heavy period. The average age at FMP for those entering menopause through surgery was 46.4 years with a range from youngest to oldest of 39 to 52. The majority of the women with hysterectomy had experienced problem periods, including symptoms of cramping, extended days of flow, heavy flows, and/or frequent intervals. Common findings for this group prior to and/or during surgery were fibroids or adhesions, and endometriosis. One of the two participants who were 52 at their last menstruations had repair of cystocele and rectocele with her total hysterectomy.

Problem Periods Leading to Hysterectomy

The youngest participant to have hysterectomy had to lobby for it. She had had two childbirths by age 21 and a tubal ligation when she was 30. In her enrollment interview, she reported she had never had PMS prior to the tubal. She was also having heavier menstrual flow and periods which lasted more days than her former pattern. She had been prescribed both pain medication for cramping and hormones to attempt to regulate her cycle. She was then 35 years old. At her Year 4 follow-up interview she reported her periods:

> continued to be absolutely horrible; cramping was horrible; the flow part was horrible. I ruined clothes and bedding. Supplywise, I couldn't believe the amount of money I was spending. I was also having hot flashes, especially in summer. I was a miserable person. I told my doctor, 'I can't deal with this any longer.'

After trying a variety of prescription medications, "My periods got worse, I was bleeding all the time with no break." Her internist referred her to a specialist for biopsy "which came back okay and I tried Provera … which just increased the problem. I had weeks of constantly bleeding and cramping." Toward her wished-for hysterectomy,

> There were certain steps we had to take because of insurance. First, I had a D&C with hysteroscopy. I woke up and said 'Is it gone?' My husband was told he [the doctor] had 'scraped a lot out.' It was growths in the uterine wall causing the cramping. The doctor reported it was 'Not cancer, but like cancer. I don't want to worry you. The only way to make it go away is to make it go away.'

The participant was relieved to finally schedule surgery.

> My ovaries, which looked to be fine, were left. At first following the hysterectomy I was depressed which I didn't expect since I was glad to have it. His nurse said it was like 'postpartum blues' and would go away which it did.

The last time this participant and I spoke was by phone for her Year 6 follow-up interview. She reported she was "doing good on no medication." She added, "Sometimes I think I have PMS in mood and water retention but not every month. Sometimes I don't have a clue till a day or two later. I don't keep a calendar." She had moved on with her life, was dealing with family matters, and some weight fluctuations.

As I've referenced previously I was challenged throughout the study as an independent researcher to keep up with the literature and attend relevant meetings. The project was consistent, continuing, and important but necessarily came after my family life and clinical career. As women in the MAPS study moved toward their final menstrual cycles, I observed several patterns I thought might prove to be significant signaling the timing of the menopause transition. In the early years, when I first began to see "double-digit" interval ranges for one year of recording, I questioned whether that represented meaningful change, but learned as time went on that some women simply had more variability to their cycles than others, which did not in itself foreshadow menopause. What was more significant was the movement of the average interval. As Treloar found, its consistent descent to a smaller number (and therefore, an increasing number of periods in one year) was associated with the onset of the menopause transition. When it grew larger again, particularly greater than 30, it generally indicated a woman was entering the later stages of the transition, shown eventually in missed months of flow. The mode was an interesting number to follow. Sometimes even as the interval range for a year seemed to vary widely, the mode remained relatively constant. The mode was what participants tended to identify as their typical experience and to plan for accordingly. Ultimately, it "dropped out"; there simply wasn't a common experience in the year, often noted by the women as unpredictable and widely variant cycles. Sometimes the disappearing mode coincided with experiencing few periods in a year's time.

Breakthrough: STRAW, ReSTAGE, and MAPS

On February 24, 2008, I emailed Dr. Lorraine Dennerstein at the University of Melbourne, Australia describing my work and interest in her book chapter "Major Findings of the Melbourne Women's Midlife Health Project" which had been referenced in an issue of *Climacteric Medicine*. I asked if it might be possible to obtain a reprint of that chapter. Dr. Dennerstein replied the same day and could not have been more kind: "I will ask my assistant to send you a list of our journal articles from our study so you can see which pdfs you would like to receive." I felt like it was Christmas in February! Her generosity allowed me a window into some very important work that had been done staging the menopause transition and a paradigm by which I could reconcile the MAPS data with internationally determined criteria.

I learned that nearly a decade after I interviewed the first participant for the MAPS project, a significant meeting of global experts from the field had been held in Utah. Among the stated objectives of the Stages of Reproductive Aging Workshop (STRAW) was the development of a useful staging system for late reproductive function. The model that emerged from STRAW identified eras of a woman's reproductive life from early reproductive through the menopausal transition to postmenopause by demarcating seven stages, five preceding and two following the FMP.

Several years following STRAW, the ReSTAGE collaboration used prospective menstrual calendar data from four cohorts (TREMIN Research Program on Women's Life, Melbourne Women's Midlife Health Project [MWMHP], Seattle Midlife Women's Health Study [SMWHS], and Study of Women's Health Across the Nation [SWAN]) to quantitatively evaluate STRAW's recommended markers for early and late menopausal transitions utilizing both menstrual calendar and endocrinological measures (Burger et al 2007, Harlow et al 2006, 2007, & Soules 2001). Whereas 80 participants had enrolled in MAPS, the four cohorts used in ReSTAGE represented significantly greater numbers. As the MAPS project moved to the conclusion of 20 years of data collection, it was quite helpful to have available the information from STRAW and ReSTAGE for guidelines evaluating project calendar data. Each of the studies which made up ReSTAGE had menstrual calendar recording as a key component which varied in design from each other and from MAPS. While none of the methods for documentation took exactly the same form (and even within the individual studies, design changes sometimes were made along the way), each had the general instruction to provide a daily record of presence (or absence) of menstrual bleeding. In turn, this information was the basis for assessing the length of bleeds, and the intervals between them.

The markers that came with STRAW followed by their further elaboration in ReSTAGE provided examples for assessing numbers from the MAPS graphs. I used the criteria from ReSTAGE publications for (1) inclusion (at least ten consecutive, nonmissing, untreated bleeding segments); (2) early transition (which I called Transition #1) "a persistent >6-day difference in consecutive cycle lengths"; and (3) late transition (Transition #2) "the occurrence of 60 or more days of amenorrhea." Following the agreed-upon convention within the field menopause was defined retrospectively as "12 months of amenorrhea following the final menstrual period (FMP)" although it was the case that a few of the women (myself included) would have another menstrual cycle years past that milestone not associated with pathology.

Given the two-decade age range at enrollment, some of the MAPS participants began recording in their data books when the criteria for the early transition already could have been met. If it was evident from the first data book, I did not count it as an official marker, since I could not verify whether it was its first occurrence for that particular person. Using this criterion, ten of the 21 women who documented an FMP in the study without the use of conventional hormones or surgical intervention recorded the early transition marker. The age range at the first transition was from 40 to 47, with a mean of 43.9 years. The range for this group of women was bimodal, including two women who enrolled in their 30s and documented a Transition #1 at age 40 and two who enrolled in their 40s and documented a Transition #1 at age 47. Allowing for the fact these numbers are too small to draw valid conclusions, my overall sense both from the data books and my conversations with the women was the Transition #1 marker was too subtle and removed from the FMP to mean much to participants unless it was accompanied by other notable changes.

In contrast, the 60 days of amenorrhea as a signpost for Transition #2 was noted by all of the women who had not had medical intervention and seemed a much more robust factor. Participants noticed missed cycles. The age range at Transition #2 was followed by the FMP at age 43 to 57, with a mean of 52.6 years. To summarize, the interval between the mean age at Transition #1 and Transition #2 was 6.2 years and between Transition #2 and the FMP 2.5 years, for an approximate 8-9 year menopause transition, also consistent with relevant literature. It was my impression that women were most keenly aware of the 3–4 years before the FMP as meaningfully different to them, described in various ways as coming close "to the end."

Flow Pattern

Flow pattern was depicted on the graph sheet by a numerical rating for any day of menstrual bleeding, as well as the total number of bleeding days in a given cycle. Similar to interval, flow range for the year was summarized from least to most number of days of flow per cycle per year; the average (mean) number of days of flow per cycle in the year; and the mode, or most frequently occurring number. Of special interest were particular bleeding patterns, such as mid-cycle flows, episodes of spotting, and number of cycles in which the participant gave a "5" for "flooding" rating, since all those experiences presented management issues to the women. As STRAW and ReSTAGE focused only on establishing interval criteria, I did not have a template with which to compare the MAPS flow patterns, although publications from different studies represented in ReSTAGE and others mentioned different aspects of flow and associated issues.

In the MAPS population, the women without the use of conventional hormone therapy or surgical interventions did not, as a group, have problematic flows. Eight of the 21 participants in this group never had a data book year with a double-digit flow range. One woman had four years of such ranges, the most in the group. For the group as a whole, so-called "run-on" periods were rare. It is also important to consider flow ratings. Many of these women were having a number of days of spotting. For some that had been usual throughout their reproductive life, but became even more pronounced as they approached their final periods. A few participants observed and recorded colored discharge or mucus which I counted because they noted it, but it was not particularly bothersome to them. The double-digit flow years often coincided with significant interval variations, the same year or close to it. In this group, "5" ratings (flooding) were rare. Often the run-on or longer cycles were near menopause, or even the FMP, noted by participants with comments such as, "I believe it is over."

Signs and Symptoms

The MAPS participants noted associated signs and symptoms with their menstrual cycles in the comments section of their data books; there were no numeric values assigned, nor a list of possible options. The observations came directly from participant experiences and their own motivation to include them. For the women who documented FMPs during the project, the signs and/or symptoms most frequently mentioned were: cramping or pain, hot flashes or night sweats, and mood shifts. The order was slightly different for those reaching a final menstrual cycle without surgical intervention or extended use of conventional hormones. In that subgroup, hot flashes or night sweats was the only sign or symptom mentioned by more than half the women, followed by cramping or pain and mood shifts. These participants appeared to note these experiences without regarding them as unduly troublesome or interfering with their functioning.

In the subgroup with surgical intervention, the most frequently noted sign or symptom was cramping or pain by 80% of the women, followed by mood shifts and insomnia or fatigue. All the participants in the subgroup who used conventional hormone therapy reported hot flashes or night sweats, followed by cramping or pain (86%) and insomnia or fatigue (71%). More than half the women in this last subgroup also reported digestive difficulties and headaches. Presumably, the more symptoms which interfered with daily life and functioning, and/or the more a given woman experienced multiple symptoms, the more likely she was to seek treatment for relief and a hoped-for return to a more satisfactory quality of life.

In 2009, I was happy to attend the Society for Menstrual Cycle Research 30th Anniversary conference in Spokane. My abstract for a paper, "Staging Menopause Applying ReSTAGE Criteria: Observations and Questions" was accepted and I had hope it would connect better with the group than had the Boulder paper in 2005. I brought my first PowerPoint slides, which were based on the deep dive into the MAPS data through Year 17. It was satisfying to be able to plug in MAPS numbers to the internationally presented paradigm and find synchrony with other, larger studies. I saw potential to achieve what participants had been aiming for: a way to locate themselves in the process.

The paper I presented was grouped under "New Research in Stages of Menopause and Perimenopause." The abstract began:

This presentation reviews briefly the rationale for staging reproductive aging, and then, discusses both challenges and opportunities for the author as she attempts to apply ReSTAGE guidelines to her own longitudinal data. Several significant studies of midlife women's health launched in the early 1990s produced meaningful information by 2001, the year of STRAW (Stages of Reproductive Aging Workshop). The ReSTAGE Collaboration followed to elaborate STRAW criteria empirically. Putting the ReSTAGE paradigm to work generates procedural questions as well as thoughts about how data which falls outside inclusion parameters can still inform the education and and treatment of midlife women.

The "inclusion criteria" referenced in the abstract had been set by ReSTAGE as "at least ten consecutive, nonmissing, untreated bleeding segments." I found this a difficult goal to achieve in the general population and felt it did not cover the full universe of menopause experience. In presenting the dilemma with questions for consideration I followed the example that had been useful to me in the Research Workshops at Georgetown: tell what you are doing, what you are wondering, and ask fellow researchers to weigh in with their own experiences, thoughts, and suggestions. The slides were a useful way not only to present basic facts about the MAPS project but to compare them with the four studies which had been part of the ReSTAGE collaboration. As I had hoped coming to the conference, this paper, which focused solely on menstrual cycle data, received more engagement from those attending than the previous one which had included concepts from family theory. Also for me the opportunity to listen to the other researchers, including their own approaches for staging information, was a gift. I returned home with renewed fervor for completing the data collection arm of the project.

In his book *How We Write*, Hilton Obenzinger (2015) reports the experience of a political scientist who took 15 years to write a book:

The first seven or eight years were spent just doing research, asking [the central] question … Research is writing: you are always taking notes …

Obenzinger shares his own process "during the dozen or more years working on this book":

Naturally, events intruded … family obligations, job demands … illness … and other excitements-and many times I had to put the book away to take

Table 4.1 Menopause Outcomes

MENOPAUSE OUTCOMES *FINAL MENSTRUAL PERIOD (FMP) documented*			
	Number of women	*Percent of FMPs documented*	*Age at FMP (Average)*
Untreated menopause (no ongoing hormone use, no surgery)	29	59%	53 years
Surgical menopause without ongoing hormone use	7	14%	46 years
Conventional hormone extensive, no surgery	4	8%	52 years
Hormone use and surgery	8	16%	46.5 years
Illness (presumed but unconfirmed breast cancer metastasis)	1	2%	48 years

FMP documented during the time of study participation.

All met ReStage criteria.

Total: 49 women of 80 enrolled.

it up again later. It was hard recalling where I was in the story, and I would have to reread (and then rewrite) the whole book each time … but these breaks did allow me to to reenter these conversations at an even deeper level, and with additional material …

For me, it was necessary to know "the end" (represented by the last of the blank books) as well as to have increased understanding of what was going on in the larger field before I could make better sense of the MAPS data. In the meantime, I wholeheartedly agree life doesn't stand still while you're waiting for your data to come in.

General Health

Participants

In the final years of the study, the remaining population had aged. Those who enrolled in their mid-30s were now nearing 50, while those who enrolled in their mid-50s were now approaching 70. I anticipated this might be reflected in their general health histories. I was aware, too, of the continuing challenge in the field about which experiences could be attributed to the end of menstrual life and which to general aging.

In the years 2008–2012, the predominant medication reported prescribed was for osteopenia or osteoporosis prevention. One woman was diagnosed with osteoarthritis in her hip and another had hip replacement. Other joint issues mentioned were "runner's knee" and shoulder pain. The next most prescribed medications were for digestive issues, hypertension, and hypothyroid. The direction of hormone therapy was reversed from earlier years of the study with more women discontinuing than adding. One participant sustained pronounced weight loss following the death of a family member while another added a medication to achieve weight loss. Other medications mentioned by just a few women were for diabetes, insomnia, anxiety, and shingles.

By far the most frequently noted category under the general question "medications and supplements" were the supplements, as women continued to self-medicate through industry trends. In addition to vitamins, Gingko biloba, CoQ10, 5-HTP, motherwort, garlic, black cohosh, and evening primrose oil were popular.

Participants who scheduled annual physicals noted cholesterol readings, and several had colon screenings. Not only polyps but also small benign tumors in other areas of the body were removed. Cataract surgeries and dental work such as crowns were mentioned. One woman reported having fallen on the ice, while another noted winter weather brought on eczema (not a new symptom for her). Another had an extended viral infection, leading to 10 days of missed work which was quite unusual for her.

Researcher

On my way to retiring from clinical practice shortly after the study concluded, I pictured the three wise monkeys: "Hear-speak-see no evil" (although in my case, symptoms emerged as speak-hear-see). In this era the hearing problem which had surfaced with a vengeance in early 2005 was less acute, partly because of adaptations I had made for it, including a variety of earplugs, noise-canceling headphones, and avoidance of crowds and noxious noise. These were strategies, not remedies. In 2010 after decades of issues with my voice, I had an evaluation for a chronic laryngitis/raw throat condition. It was becoming increasingly difficult to make myself heard by the automated answering systems of insurance companies without further straining my voice. Thankfully the evaluation revealed no structural problems but I again received advice to better manage my allergies and asthma. Two sessions with a speech pathologist were also useful. I learned compensations I had made to try to lessen the problem were in fact intensifying it, a lesson which I'd met in other areas of my life and a reminder of the question from Thich Nhat Hanh, "Are you sure?"

A year following the voice evaluation, the most worrisome and disruptive physical symptom surfaced. In the summer of 2011, I was attempting to load MAPS data into a spreadsheet and experiencing trouble locating the cursor. Repeatedly I would shut my right eye to see more clearly. I figured I needed new glasses and saw my long-time optometrist who shocked me by saying, "You need to see a retina specialist within a week." Luckily, he knew just the person. With my husband and good friends providing support and transportation, I had a vitrectomy in September of that year. One of the side effects of such surgery is the growth or development of pre-existing cataracts. The cataract in my right eye which had begun as "age-appropriate" to be monitored galloped away after the surgery. In 2012 I had another surgery in the same eye. That eye had been dominant and the continuing loss of central vision created a problem re-establishing binocular vision. My brain didn't know which eye to believe, creating occasional double vision that I could blink out of when I realized what was happening. Over the next few years, I had cataract surgery in the left eye also and eventually YAG-laser treatment in each eye for posterior capsule opacification (PCO). This totaled five procedures in five years. After each one, I would think maybe things would improve sufficiently to consider driving on the highway but after brief attempts, I ultimately realized that wouldn't be possible. It put me in a novel position needing help, when I was used to thinking of myself as the helper. At the same time, I was always aware of all the people in the world suffering with conditions much more dire than mine and without benefit of the supports I had. Mindfulness meditation from the Plum Village tradition was a key for keeping proper perspective, managing medical situations and daily life, while cultivating gratitude for good health overall.

Family Relationships

Participants

In the final years of the project, one woman married her long-time partner, while a couple of participants reported challenges in their long-time marriages. Another woman divorced her second husband after 17 years of marriage. They had married in the early years of the project. Overall, in this era there was more focus on health issues as well as retirement plans for husbands. As one would expect, there were no pregnancies or births reported for these older age participants, and no menarche ages reported for their daughters either. Instead reports centered on educational milestones and marriages for their children and the births of 14 grandchildren by 10 participants, as well as the adoption of a grandchild for another participant. This highly educated group of women seemed to produce well-educated children as well, including those with advanced professional degrees.

Two women experienced the deaths of their mothers and two the deaths of their fathers. Six participants reported illnesses and/or serious surgeries for their parents sometimes requiring a period of caregiving at home or in a facility. Family stressors could accumulate: a participant and her husband, both only children in their original families, experienced the diagnosis of macular degeneration for her mother and the deaths of her father and his mother, all within a couple of years. Another woman reported the deaths of both her parents three months apart followed by the death of an older sister at the age of 60 from a brain tumor. Participants also continued to note the deaths of important aunts and uncles.

Each addition or subtraction from the family system by birth, marriage, divorce, or death leads to a re-ordering, either great or small, within the larger group. For designated caregivers within the family there can be a particularly heavy burden of tasks and responsibilities; conversely, other members with different functional roles can feel left out of important decision-making, such as choices for an ill parent or distribution of property following a death. The families of participants represented a continuum from groups who communicated and cooperated well in times of transition to those whose relationships fractured and were not repaired, with every gradation in between.

20-Year Review of Family Relationship Facts for MAPS Participants

Partners

All told for the length of the study, the relationship status of the great majority (55 of 80 women) continued without change during their time in the project given the differential participation from baseline to the 22 who stayed 20 years.

Eleven women married during the study, including three who married long-time partners. Twelve were divorced from their husbands in marriages as brief as four years or as long as 29. Five lesbian women had enrolled in the research study, including two cohabiting couples. The fifth, single at enrollment, lived with her partner early in the project during a relationship which ended within two years. The two same-sex couples at enrollment broke up after three and eighteen years together respectively. Another participant married her same-sex partner in a civil ceremony several years after divorcing her husband. A woman who divorced her first husband after 24 years married her second six years later. They too divorced after 17 years. Two women were widowed during the research study at the rather young ages of 47 and 52 respectively, one due to the illness of her husband and the other to accident.

Children

The breadth of our study and the age span of participants at enrollment offered the opportunity to sketch a full generation of development for their children. Eighteen women documented the menarche ages for their daughters in real time while 21 reported the birth of at least one grandchild during their project participation. Seventy percent of study participants who were mothers reported significant educational milestones for their children ranging from high school diplomas to PhD and MD degrees. The remaining mothers had young children at the time of their project participation. Twenty-three women noted marriages for their children, two of whom divorced.

Parents

Ten of the participants had experienced the deaths of both parents prior to their enrollment in the study, but were not necessarily in the oldest age groups enrolling. Thirty-seven women experienced the deaths of parents during the study, including ten for whom this was their first parent to die, sometimes leaving a surviving parent needing care and attention. Seven of the women were orphaned during the time of their project participation. One participant, whose birth mother died when she was an infant and whose father had died

Table 4.2 Family Transitions Recorded for the 20-Year Participants

FAMILY TRANSITIONS RECORDED FOR THE 20-year participants during the study

AGE AT ENROLLMENT
BY INTERVAL
(Number of women participating 20 years)

34–39   (6)
40–44   (10)
45–49   (5)
50–55   (1)
TOTAL: 22 OF 80 who enrolled

PARTNER TRANSITIONS

No primary relationship change	Divorces, 3 who remarried	Married and widowed	Remained single-no change	TOTAL:
15	5	1	1	22

PARENT PARTICIPANT DEATH

Both parents died	Both parents are still living	Last living parent died	Mother died	Father died	Bio father died before study
8	2	8	1	2	1

prior to her enrollment, experienced during the project the death of her step-mother, the person who had been her functional mother all of her recalled life.

Researcher

In 2008 my mother's entire immediate family, with the exception of my niece's husband, were able to gather at her home for her 85th birthday. By then, she had two great-grandchildren, my first grandchild born the previous year and my sister's born eight months afterward. This echoed the situation for their mothers (our daughters) who had been born eight months apart 27 years earlier. Price-less pictures were taken to commemorate the occasion, which stands as the last time Mom was able to enjoy being with all of us at the same time, although she eventually lived to be 94 and had two additional great-grandchildren and another on the way at the time of her death in 2018. My sister and her husband continued to visit regularly as usual, but as our children grew, gradu-ated, had jobs, married, and had their own children, it seemed the country grew, too, and trips from the western states were challenging to coordinate. For the most part, my husband and I were able to make at least annual trips to see our daughter and her family and provide financial assistance for them to visit us, and therefore, Mom. This pattern echoed how Mom had visited my sister's family during her many years of widowhood, and she and my dad while he was liv-ing. Another generation back, it was similar to the situations of visits with my father's parents. My mother's family rarely visited the Midwest, so we kept in contact by other means. At the Celebration of Life for Mom, her grandchildren each spoke to the very personal relationships they had had with her despite the miles. In addition to phone calls, as technology advanced, there had been emails as well as Mom's primary reason for being on Facebook!

A couple of months before our granddaughter's birth my husband and I had purchased a mini-motorhome which facilitated the round trips. We enjoyed the beautiful country and national parks on the way for several years and a number of visits. We took our first plane trip to Montana for our grand-son's birth in late November 2012. Given my continuing vision problems, my mother's increasing needs, and the expense to maintain the Rialta, we sold it the following year.

Through these years, Mom and I evaluated the resources available to help her continue to manage in her own home and respect her choice for as much independence as possible. She applied for a handicapped parking permit for the use of her various drivers, and in 2010, we realized a wearable call button would be a good idea. As her first contact on the emergency system, I entered the era of 24-7 on-call. Step by step Mom turned over manage-ment of her financial affairs to me. Since she was the one from whom I had learned money management in the first place, our views were quite compat-ible. We kept my sister informed for major decisions and consulted her when questions arose. A child of the Depression, Mom conserved very frugally the funds she received related to my father's early death when she was in her 50s, but as the years passed, those resources decreased while her in-home help needs increased. This created anxiety for both of us and I consulted the elder care attorney who had handled Mom's will and also advised my husband's family during his parents' aging years. I was very grateful Mom, my sister, and I could communicate well about the challenges and knew not to take that gift for granted.

In the final years of the research study, my father-in-law's medical condition including both lung and heart issues was punctuated by acute crises necessitating hospitalization and consideration of how long he and his significant other could manage on their own. I recall one of the times my husband and I along with his sister and her husband were called in the middle of the night to come to the hospital. Studying our faces in the waiting area I thought, "We're not so young either." Pop's last move with his partner was back to a private residence, next door to one of her daughters. In the fall of 2010 he had an episode requiring a relatively brief time on life support, but it was followed by the final one in January 2011. At that time, the four of us were called to make the decision to remove him from support. My sister-in-law asked the attending physician, "If this was your father what would you do?" To all of us this time seemed qualitatively different and it was our family consensus according to medical advice to "let him go." I am grateful for how lucky my husband and I were to have such uncomplicated relationships with both our sisters and their husbands as our parents aged and faced their variety of challenges. Commemorative ceremonies and the settling of estates which followed were also managed with a cooperative spirit and little fuss, which I knew from all my interviews with clients and research participants was not always the case.

Life Situation: Career, Education, and Geographic Moves

Participants

Just one participant in the final years mentioned she had begun school toward a new career. She was one of the younger women when she enrolled in her 30s, had several geographic moves, all in the same general area, and several job changes during the time of the project. This career shift marked a transition from work in the business sector to a service profession. Through all the changes, she presented as a self-motivated person who functioned well as an independent practitioner. At the same time her family life had relative stability, her friendship base was strong, and she had made a number of thoughtful decisions about how much volunteer community work to do.

Seven participants noted job changes during the final years, including promotions in their usual fields. One woman's marital separation coincided with both a geographic move and change in office location. The following year she and her husband divorced. Job and/or relationship changes led to geographic moves for two other women. For most of the participants remaining in the

Decision-Making

Hysterectomy was warranted because fibroid was so large it was crowding other organs. The surgery wasn't a big deal overall. They found endometriosis everywhere, lots of scar tissue from a previous procedure on my colon. I decided not to have ovaries; it's not in the family, but two people I know had ovarian cancer. They also took the cervix so that is three kinds of cancer I don't have to worry about now. If my dad hadn't been sick, I might have done this sooner. I knew, 'This doesn't seem right.'

About three months ago, the bottom dropped out. I was having very heavy periods close together. I am scheduled for a hysterectomy two weeks from today. I thought, 'I am not going to deal with this. Primary care doctor referred me to a gynecologist. I have tried drugs and was not interested in being on long-term medication. My blood pressure was a factor. We talked some about a D & C, but might just need something else later. Fibroids are what I have. It happened kind of fast. I feel healthy, upbeat. I never gave a thought to childbearing.

Primary care doctor talked to me about hormone therapy. I don't know if I want to go on it. The more I read the more confused I get so I think, 'Stop reading!' The doctor is pushing it strongly. I don't think all women are the same.

The tubal ligation was right after the second birth. I went to have a baby and came out with the tubal. I was 31. The doctor tried to argue with me, but I said, 'Do I look like a person who changes my mind?'

I have made some clear decisions. I changed doctors from the get-go. I have to be in charge. I respect this woman. I got a script for hormones but refused to take it. Regard it as an 'insurance policy'. I don't have hot flashes. Everybody has skin stuff. The blood test showed estradiol was down. There is no reason for me to take hormone replacement. I do my Kegels. I'm not doing the maximum of everything I can do. I had a period of time I was totally crazy-difficulty with my parents, changes at work. Since Christmas I have been a lot better. I made the determination I could only do so much with my parents.

final years, the era was characterized by stability and less change than in previous years.

Researcher

My vision problems brought to a head the feasibility of continuing a solo private practice in which insurance billing was done increasingly through electronic means. I also typed my own clinical notes and had never had employees. As my 65th birthday approached in 2012, my husband and I consulted with our financial planner and I made the decision to close my clinical practice in January 2013. This followed the final MAPS interviews in the fall of 2012. Having heard horror stories of therapists who "took off" without preparing their clients, I was grateful to be able to plan well in advance with mine toward the end of my practice and facilitate referrals to other providers for those who desired them. I notified insurance companies and other professional organizations of my target date for retirement and felt lighter doing so.

While I was preparing to leave clinical work, I was devoting increasing time to teaching meditation in the community and pursuing ordination in the Order of Interbeing in Plum Village tradition (the tradition of Thich Nhat Hanh). In the spring of 2012 at a retreat in Omaha the visiting dharma teacher suggested in a personal interview I could begin a sangha (mindfulness meditation practice group) in my home town. After first brainstorming with another social worker who had attended one of my first community classes and continued with the meditation group that followed, an organizing committee was formed in the summer of 2012. On September 7, 2012 Deep Listening Sangha of Lawrence held its first practice. Until my mother's needs precluded it, I continued to offer classes in the community at a variety of venues. It seemed there was cross-fertilization between the more Buddhist-based sangha, the more secular community classes, the closure of the data collection arm of the research study, and clinical retirement.

Friends, Volunteer Work, and Community Activities

Questions related to participants' friendship groups, volunteer and other community activities were not a formal part of the standard interview process throughout the years of the study but these interactions and commitments were routinely mentioned by the women and are represented in my interview notes. Female friendships, in particular, were an important resource for participants coping with multiple demands on time and energy and health care decisions. Since siblings were a natural part of the family diagram, I noted the rewarding contacts many of the women had with their sisters. For participants whose mothers had died or were no longer able to communicate, sisters could fill the gap by providing a listening ear, reference point for experiences, and support.

A number of the women typically included their voluntary community activities when I asked for life situation updates. These could be church-related, or secular at the local, regional, or state levels. As participants weighed just how much time and energy they had available for pursuits outside work and family, sometimes they increased community participation and other times found they needed to cutback. Like friendships, the relationship systems accompanying these activities, when they went smoothly, could provide a nice balance to the more complex and emotionally weighted relationships with family members and colleagues.

References

Burger, H.G., Hale, G. E., Robertson, D.M., & Dennerstein, L. (2007). A review of hormonal changes during the menopausal transition: focus on findings from the Melbourne Women's Midlife Health Project. *Human Reproduction Update* 13(6):559–565. https://doi.org/10.1093/humupd/dmm020

Harlow, S.D., Cain, K., Crawford, S., Dennerstein, L., Little, R., Mitchell, E.S., Bin Nan, Randolph, J.F. Jr., Taffe, J., &Yosef, M. (2006). Evaluation of four proposed bleeding criteria for the onset of late menopausal transition. *The Journal of Endocrinology & Metabolism* 91(9):3432–3438. https://doi.org/10.1210/jc.2005-2810

Harlow, S.D., Crawford, S., Dennerstein, L., Burger, H.G., Mitchell, E.S., & Sowers, M.F. (2007). Recommendations from a multi-study evaluation of proposed criteria for staging reproductive aging. *Climacteric* 10:112–119. https://doi.org/10.1080/13697130701258838

Obenzinger, H. (2015). *How we write: The varieties of writing experience*. CreateSpace Independent Publishing Platform. ISBN-13: 978-1517152604.

Soules, M.R., Sherman, S., Parrott, E., Rebar, R., Santoro, N., Utian, W., & Woods, N. (2001). Executive summary: Stages of reproductive aging workshop (STRAW). *Fertility and Sterility* 76(5):874–878. https://doi.org/10.1016/s0015-0282(01)02909-0

Part 2

The Study of Change Over Time

Having presented the history of the research project by eras in Part 1, Part 2 moves on to the discussion phase of what was learned and introduces the Multiple Continuum Assessment as a useful tool for contemplating the menopause transition as an ongoing life process in context. The value and possibilities of longitudinal work are emphasized.

DOI: 10.4324/9781003540830-6

5　Project Strengths and Limitations

Women do not go through the menopause transition in a vacuum. Their experience exists in a web of relationships with family, friends, work, educational systems, communities, and society at large. Based on the menstrual cycle research of Dr. Alan Treloar and the multigenerational family research of Dr. Murray Bowen, participants in this project charted their menstrual cycles in data books until the time of their FMP. Family, health, and life situation information was updated annually using a family diagram, personal interviews, and questionnaires. The study validated stages of the menopausal transition against the backdrop of the stages of family life at a particular time in history. Also documented were the varieties of decisions project participants made to cope with the changes in their bodies and ongoing lives. The women who stayed many years in the project reported how useful data collection was to them and the 1:1 method of interviews confirmed their experience. Although a relatively homogeneous sample, the study demonstrated the uniqueness of each woman's experience and the importance of life context. The longitudinal design of the project highlighted the dynamic quality of life over time.

The boundaries of the MAPS study were identified at the beginning, although it grew tenfold from two years to twenty. The framework was a two-prong approach of recording menstrual cycles and updating family diagram, health, and life history annually. It was not a randomized trial; participants entered the study as what is known as a "convenience sample" and left of their own accord, when (1) they had gone as far as they wished, by personal interest and/or availability; (2) "graduated" by documenting their FMPs; or (3) reached project end when the last blank data book was exchanged the fall of 2012.

While the study group seemed uniform demographically, by report the participants ran the gamut of menopausal experience. Because of the age range at enrollment, the longitudinal format allowed a close-eyed view of variation not only from woman to woman but within the experience of individuals over time. This underscored the limitations of "snapshot" studies which capture and possibly overdramatize particular moments in time and miss the nuances of ongoing processes. It was especially helpful to have 22 participants opt to remain past the "blank book" to provide postmenopausal data.

DOI: 10.4324/9781003540830-7

I was not thinking in terms of independent and dependent variables in constructing the MAPS design, as I assumed interlocking variables. It began and remained an observational study exploring a natural system in process. I didn't view the participants and their experiences in isolation, but as part of multiple overlapping relationship networks. Although the project began with the proposal of a two-year pilot, I was aware from the start of the value of longitudinal study, from Dr. Treloar's own work documenting menstrual cycles as well as Dr. Bowen's with multigenerational families (Treloar 1967, Bowen & Butler 2013, Noone 2024). Many studies in the natural world as well as research labs demonstrate the learning available by viewing change over time Mitchell (2012). Surprises occur that could not have been predicted and might have been missed in short interval work. Through longitudinal, systems-based study, a wide-angle long lens is available which can put developments in context with what came before and what followed (Friedman & Martin 2012, Nesselroade & Baltes 1979). That said, with its base of prospective recording, MAPS was always grounded in the present moment.

Cognition, Emotionality, and Spiritual Well-Being

One of the thoughts that was scary to me about menopause was not being able to think. I have noticed the opposite.

Episodes of anxiety, unclear thinking, can be pretty intense. Three weeks ago after a movie at night when I left theater, I felt like I was on acid or something. Didn't know where I was. Wondered should I pull over, say to these kids, "I'm going to call somebody to get us home."

Started running again in June. Have always walked. Aerobic capacity is still there. Complete miracle, never expected to run again. Diet changed because it does; food that will fuel it better. Never expected to feel so good when I was nearly 52 years old. Has been kind of transforming in a spiritual way, even more important to me than the physical. Thirty-year meditation anniversary yesterday. Sat just thinking, following my own thoughts, started writing later in the day. Have found myself wanting to read more philosophy. Just want to know more.

It has not been twelve consecutive months yet. Do feel pretty free and clear of it. Do believe there's still a hormonal uproar. Days angry from the get-go. Did back out of an alley and ran into a lady's car on a day like that. Not having the stupid time things like I did for a while.

I have been reading as much as I can. Last year short-term memory loss. Could be my attention to it. Times I cannot track: 'You have to say that to me again.' That's unsettling to me. Can put up with the crazy cycles, night sweats around menstrual flow itself.

Don't feel so groggy-headed as I did for a while. Walk at 5 a.m., yoga at night.

> One month no flow at all. Surprise to me. Was feeling pretty premenstrual. Waiting and waiting and nothing happened. Out of the blue around Thanksgiving, didn't expect. I had been planning a trip-incredible lethargy and stuckness, got my period. Had been so out of the loop didn't think that could be the reason. Was actually missing it – want to do a ceremony and mourn it. Was talking to someone who was so excited to be finishing her periods. Not so much missing the low; but feeling so even all the time. Used to have a day I felt invincible.

Insofar as I am aware this study stands alone in its systematic recording of menstrual cycle, health, family, and life situation information simultaneously over time. It does not include specific biomedical measures nor confirmation with sources other than the women themselves. The project benefited and suffered in ways typical of longitudinal studies. The chief benefit was the advantage of observing a physiological process and family events through many years. Guesses emerged almost immediately as to what constituted temporary change and what might be the "crossed line" into menopause. These guesses were formulated in my own mind and some data searching as the principal investigator, but also by the women in their own lived lives hoping to locate themselves in the process. As time went by, patterns were seen and hypotheses refined. For some what had seemed like sharp changes gradually softened and ebbed away. For others sharpness was the central organizing principle, before and after hysterectomy for example. Even that direct variation had different looks for different participants: old symptoms resolved, new symptoms occurring, and necessary adjustments along the way. The length and breadth of the study design naturally invited the concept of continuum and put the menopause transition in its proper place, neither center stage nor background.

The chief research challenge was unplanned variation in recording: missed months not by evidence or lack of menstruation but by forgetting or miscategorizing experience. Personal interviews served as opportunities for clarification, as well as the continuing relationship development between researcher and participant. The fact I was the sole contact person for the project carried the advantage of familiarity and continuity of method, but introduced the possibility of blind spots and unchecked perceptions. As a midlife woman myself going through similar experiences to the participants, there was a natural base from which to relate and a useful language. I maintained throughout the project that each woman's journey was uniquely her own as the only person living in her body while I remained curious and open to her views and choices. I believe the natural camaraderie that developed was more helpful than not in promoting our mutual interest in the data. Seeing with "systems eyes" helped me consider each woman in context from the beginning and solidified with the initial construction of her family diagram. I never forgot she was connected to the family from which she came, the people with whom she lived and worked during the time of the study, and other situations in which she made commitments and spent time and energy. I was aware from my clinical work that listening to one member of a relationship represents only that person's unique perspective and others in the same system may hold different views.

Project participants expressed that the recording process and the personal follow-up interviews allowed them to consider their experiences more objectively, and interact with their health providers around real-time data. The presence of the diagram in our interviews and questions consistently tailored to include "the rest of life" offered the opportunity to consider the whole of their experience in a reflective and non-pressured way. Many of the women commented that simply being listened to by someone outside their normal circle of relationships in a focused but relaxed and supportive atmosphere was unusual in their lives. They expressed it helped them to think through what was happening to them less judgmentally as well, with more interest and less urgency, and to feel less alone.

References

Bowen, M., & Butler, J. (2013). *The origins of family psychotherapy: The NIMH Family Study Project.* Lanham, MD: Jason Aronson.

Friedman, H.S., & Martin, L.R. (2012). *The longevity project: Surprising discoveries for health and long life from the landmark eight-decade study.* Plume. ISBN-13: 978-0452297708.

Mitchell, S. (2012). *Unsimple truths: Science, complexity, and policy.* Chicago: The University of Chicago Press. ISBN-13:978–0226006628.

Nesselroade, J.R., & Baltes, P. B. (1979). *Longitudinal research in the study of behavior and development.* New York: Academic Press. ISBN-13: 978-0125156608.

Noone, R. (2024). From the editor. *Family Systems: A Journal of Natural Systems Thinking in Psychiatry and the Sciences* 18:2 Washington, DC: The Bowen Center for the Study of the Family. https://www.thebowencenter.org/journal

Treloar, A.E., Boynton, R.E., Behn, B.G., & Brown, B. W. (1967). Variation of the human menstrual cycle through reproductive life. *International Journal of Fertility* 12(1 Pt 2):77–126.

6   Life in Context

Depicting and Living with Change

From the beginning, I wished to place a study of the menopause transition within the circumstances of the participants' lives as they unfolded. This fit with my career as a social worker, my education and training within family theory, and my own life experience. Reviewing the literature I had been put off by the way in which women's lives were divided: now we are discussing their periods, now we are taking up their medical histories, now and then we may give a mention to their families or to the cultures in which they reside. I knew, instinctively and by observation, that all these elements influenced and were influenced by each other. There was no actual separation that would hold up on closer inspection.

When I was a medical social worker on a dialysis unit in Denver, staff signaled that one of our patients, who was diabetic and actually doing well medically as far as lab values and other measures were concerned, seemed to be depressed. When I spoke with her, I learned she was at the age her mother had been when the mother died. It seemed useful to her to voice the history and be heard, so she could then engage and be pleased with her own present-day progress. That was but one example of the connections I could see that went beyond numbers, and this was after having taken one course on family in graduate school, but before formal training in family theory and therapy. When I was introduced to the concepts of Bowen Theory, I acquired names for phenomena I had observed (and participated in all my life in my own family).

Navigating the Medical System

Horrible year of sleeping. Went to see a psychiatrist in January to get a light box on referral from my doctor. He determined in a very short time that he thought I was bipolar. Prescribed Tegritol – at the time I was just happy he gave me a script. Then thought, "Wait a minute. I just agreed to take medication that can damage my liver." He did give me information about light box on second visit. Decided Premarin had a real chemical feel and replaced it with 2 mg Estradiol. Seems to help

---

DOI: 10.4324/9781003540830-8

sleeping. Appointment scheduled to see gynecologist I've heard good things about.

My philosophy is: if not broke, don't fix it. Minor things occur; I think "need to walk" – will cure it.

Seeing a general practitioner now. The experience I had with the OB-GYN was really negative … None of them on their own came to the conclusion maybe some blood tests in order. Because I was so young. First thing when I had the blood test run the doctor said, "I'm writing you a prescription for estrogen." I said, "I'm open to the possibility that may be the only thing that works, but I know estrogen makes me depressed. I want to try something else first." He said okay.

Used to take progesterone twice a day, she combined with estriol. Thinking about going off altogether after WHI. Hard for me to talk with her, so evangelical. We compromised – taking once a day instead.

Insurance company tried to become doctor saying I couldn't have a certain medication. Pills $10 a pill. Doctor got so mad. "I'll take care of it." Not doing the HRT, doing really well. Have been sleeping also. That's been important.

Had car accident last year. Had to talk with medical examiner; he would have loved to have labeled me "problems because of menopause" – I told him I had been in this for 11 years.

Temporary use of birth control pills really makes things easier for those of us who are hikers. General health great, iron okay. Allergy medication PRN in May.

In the 1980s my first doctor (male) said I needed a hysterectomy for fibroids, but second doctor (female) said no.

Continuum is defined as "a coherent whole characterized as a collection, sequence, or progression of values or elements varying by minute degrees." Now looking up the word (concept) I am interested to learn its origin is derived from the Latin "continuous." Its first usage is noted in the 1700s, with a swift uptick about the year of my birth, 1947 (Merriam-Webster, n.d.). By the time I came to family systems theory in my 30s, the concept of continuum was familiar to me and I could naturally accept its central importance to Dr. Bowen's thinking. Earlier I had had the experience in graduate school in which one of my mentors pointed out "you can take any continuum and turn it into a dichotomy" which had already given me a different perspective on the black-white binary common to our human brains.

Differentiation of self is a central tenet of Bowens theory which Daniel Papero et al. (2018) have described as a continuum of variation. I find shifting focus to continuum opens to a wider perspective; a breath of fresh air more representative of reality. I came to use continuum thinking in my clinical work considering the diagnoses required by insurance companies. I realized behaviors identified as "bipolar disorder" are not actually an "either-or" proposition. We all experience variations in mood and energy levels, without necessarily crossing an arbitrary line to pathology. Similarly, while humans vary in the extent to which they manifest what Bowen termed solid self, it is not the case that some of us are 100% differentiated and some are zero (Frost in Keller & Noone, 2020).

More than a Number

Because of the continuing flow of life in varied directions, characterizing categories of experience as numerical values can be a bit of a trap which turns ongoing hypotheses into slices or snapshots. For the MAPS data, including the proposed Multiple Continuum Assessment, I find trajectories and co-occurrence of interrelated variables to be more informative than the assignment of numbers along a scale. Observations made over time capture fluidity not available by short-term study. In his Foreword to the *Handbook of Bowen Family Systems Theory and Research Methods* (Keller & Noone, 2020) Michael Kerr states, "An absence of mathematical models is not a reason for family researchers to get defensive," and points out "Bowen described myriad functional facts of family interactions gleaned from extensive observational research," which eventually led to the basic concepts of his theory. Early in my study of the theory, I remember hearing Dr. Bowen say on more than one occasion, "You can't chi square a feeling and make it a fact."

"Bell Curve" of a Transition: Depicting Change

Dr. Bowen wrote that "The continuum of basic levels of differentiation for our species seems to be a bell-shaped curve." He called it a "continuum of adaptiveness" (Bowen, 1978).

When charting a transition, in addition to its horizontal axis, a vertical movement over time also depicts context in an individual's life. Eighty women enrolled during 1991–1992. As noted in the Early Years chapter, the one participant who died during the time of her participation in the project was a young woman whose breast cancer had been diagnosed soon after childbirth and prior to her enrollment. She did not choose follow-up treatment after surgery and whether or not for that reason became the exception to the overall theme of the midlife era in the MAPS group: survival and adaptation. The 20 years of data collection told the story of experiencing changes and dealing with them.

With nonsurgical ("natural") menopause, the picture, if not the math, of a bell curve does indeed come to mind. The menstrual cycle data advanced slowly over the years from subtle to noteworthy difference, and then eased out toward the postmenopause during the year in which the Final Menstrual

Period was documented. Younger-enrolling participants who withdrew prior to documenting visible changes in their cycles often noted shifts in other areas of their lives. The oldest-enrolling participants sometimes had already experienced their most pronounced menstrual cycle changes but those who continued to participate for the length of the study reported what came after in the way of health, family, and general adjustment to aging. Since the majority of those at enrollment were in their early 40s, the largest capture of the study was the perimenopause, which, not coincidentally, was also the era of most notable change.

Uncertainty

In the recent book *Musings on Perimenopause and Menopause: Identity, Experience, Transition* (Dillaway & Wershler, 2021), Dillaway, contributes a chapter titled, "Waiting for Seventeen Days." She comments

> Having studied menopause and reproductive aging for almost two decades, and having no other reason to miss a period that month, and having already experienced some early signs of perimenopause, I knew the reason my period was late … But having a forty-seven-day cycle out of the blue was like being thrown off course, forced to miss the thirty-day mark my body and I were used to.

She links her experience in a multigenerational context, having anticipated using a period-tracking app with her teenage daughter right after the daughter's menarche, as well as remembering her own mother's menopause experience:

> My daughter has come to understand that both our menstrual lives are shifting, mine winding down while hers winds up. At least we have this shift in common … I remember how frazzled and uncertain [my mother] … seemed about her changes … Only now do I begin to understand how she must have felt about the uncertainty.

For women with significant symptoms having hysterectomy, the slow and subtle climb to the bell curve's peak may have been co-opted by the urgency of events. There, the uncertainty rests in making a decision on hearing a surgeon's recommendation and not knowing the ultimate result, either for findings or resolution of problems. There are also questions of how involved the surgery will be and whether hormone treatment postprocedure will also be recommended. Generally, the physician will review with the participant (as patient) her expectations but also require a release prior to the procedure which could include more extensive or invasive work.

Participants following the path of beginning differences in interval and/or flow as well as signs and symptoms signaling perimenopause progressing to the final menstrual period and beyond, have had colorful ways to describe the movement from predictable to unpredictable cycles. Our year-by-year interviews presented the chance to track this development in real time.

A woman who enrolled at age 40 said in her Year 8 follow-up,

> Everything was pretty much the same except in August I was a week and a half late and thought, "Oh, no, pregnant." Not having a period would not bother me but I don't want the symptoms of menopause … My feeling was [there was] some connection between stresses at the time and the late period.

The following year she reported,

> Having longer intervals now; this month I was 10 days late which has happened twice this year. I have found feeling like a period is starting and then not kind of yucky. Twice I went out and got pregnancy tests. Bloated, headache, don't feel energetic. Change in my life is affecting my cycle, but overall I feel a lot more calm.

She summarized in Year 10, "The movement to menopause basically seems like a slow process which is fine with me. I remember one or two years ago I felt bad when I was supposed to be starting, [this year] I haven't noticed that." In the next annual review she expressed, "It would be nice to be done," and after documenting her final menstrual period in Year 14, she reported, "Having no flow is a lot simpler." She enjoyed having "thrown out all my yucky underwear." The big news that year was the birth of her first grandchild.

This participant's account through the years highlights several themes of the perimenopause: the movement from "expected" to "whenever" (as another woman phrased it); the pregnancy concern in the absence of the usual pattern; the sensations that can occur when the body seems to be gearing up for the usual cycle and then doesn't complete it; the hypothesizing that goes on to make sense of changes, often in the context of concurrent shifts in other areas of life; and the overall relief (the downslope on the bell curve) reaching the new era.

In her book, *Call Them by Their True Names* (2018), author Rebecca Solnit states, "Accommodating change and uncertainty requires a looser sense of self, an ability to respond in various ways … It begins with being open to the possibilities and interested in the complexities." Even after the final period is confirmed and women have expressed their elation "being done," they can simultaneously be caught up short with symptoms like hot flashes and night sweats which continue long past what they might have expected. The privilege of continuing the study into postmenopause led to the identification of other curves in which something like hot flashes can move from "nothing at all disturbing" to "very intense; I was hoping I'd be through all that" to "haven't noticed."

The women who opted for natural menopause mentioned being aware there were treatment options but hadn't crossed the line to thinking they were necessary. Often the marker was how intrusive they found various signs and symptoms in their daily lives, as well as how much space they had in coping to regard them as "interesting," as Solnit says. Dillaway and Wershler (2021) write,

> Uncertainties can be unsettling and unpleasant as we live through and with them. Questioning whether one is perimenopausal or menopausal, for instance, is an uncomfortable feeling … waiting for periods is hard enough, let alone waiting to see if one has had their final period … Instead of allowing master narratives to define who they are, women can embrace their uncertainties and interpret their transitions more personally. Perhaps this means we need to consider that women's feelings of flux, duality and uncertainty are not only normal and natural but necessary during this reproductive transition. Maybe this is true through reproductive lives in general … authors in this volume also affirm that unique life contexts and connections to others may determine more of women's individual experience than the biological or physiological bases of reproductive aging.

The Useful Limit of "Stage"

The concept of stage is familiar in our society as well as to scholars in research. The assumption of stage is a passage, coming from something and presumed to be moving to something else. My first introduction to this view in a memorable way came during graduate school listening to Elisabeth Kubler-Ross (1974, 2014). She had lit a fire of discussion in the health and mental health fields with her "stages of dying." As I began to read about menopause in the context of reproductive life there was a reference to the Tanner Stages (Cleveland Clinic, 2024) as another system of physical development. Stages can be an extremely helpful way to categorize experience and locate oneself and others in time, habit, and expectation. The problem comes when our brains carry them too far by assuming that all people travel through them in a similar way, or that (depending on the subject matter) stages are always taken in order. This was a concern of Kubler-Ross who later in her career emphasized she simply meant to capture universal possibilities for reacting to the end of life, not a schedule for doing it "right."

As I mentioned in Chapter 4, efforts by reproductive researchers in STRAW and ReSTAGE were a breakthrough for me in analyzing data from the MAPS project. The seven stages first sketched in STRAW were a manageable number to which the people passing through them, the physicians treating them, and the researchers studying the process could easily relate. But I realized along the way that sometimes the idea could be taken too far with nearly every change labeled "stage." In a publication "Staging the Menopausal Transition:

Data from the Tremin Research Program on Women's Health" Mansfield and her colleagues (2004) concluded:

> Women do not all follow one orderly progression from pre- to peri- to postmenopause. It is true that the majority of women did so, stopping along the way for varying numbers of year at each stage. But others flip-flopped between stages, and still others reached menopause and then resumed menstrual bleeding. Some women remained at a stage for years, others did not. Some women had long transitions, others did not. At least one woman reached menopause following a menstrual life of regularity, with no noticeable changes observed. A similar pattern was observed by McKinlay, Brambilla, and Posner (1992) who found that 10% of their participants ceased menstruating abruptly with little to no perimenopausal irregularity.

The value of the longitudinal study with interviews was to record not only actual flow, signs, and symptoms, but also the accompanying sense of time passing and each person's unique experience within it.

References

Bowen, M. (1978). *Family therapy in clinical practice*. New York: Jason Aronson. ISBN: 0-087668-334-0.

Cleveland Clinic (2024-last reviewed) Puberty: Tanner Stages for Boys and Girls. https://myclevelandclinic.org/health/body/puberty.

Dillaway, H. & Wershler, L., Eds. (2021). *Musings on perimenopause and menopause: Identity, experience, transition*. Bradford, Ontario, Canada: Demeter Press. ISBN-13: 978-1772582857.

Keller, M.N. & Noone, R.J. Eds. (2020). *Handbook of Bowen Family Systems Theory and research methods: A systems model for family research*. New York and Abington: Routledge. ISBN: 978-1-138-47812-1.

Kubler-Ross, E. (1974, 2014). *On death and dying: What the dying have to teach doctors, nurses, clergy, and their own families*. Scribner Reissue edition. ISBN-13: 978-14766775548.

McKinlay, S.M., Brambilla, D.I., & Posner, J.G. (1992). *The normal menopause transition. Maturitas 14*(2):103-15. https//doi.org/10.1016/0378-5122 (92) 90003-m.

Mansfield, P., Carey, M., Anderson, A., Barsom, S., & Koch, P. (2004). Staging the menopausal transition: Data from the Tremin Research Program on Women's Health. *Women's Health Issues* 14(6). Washington, DC. Jacobs Institute of Women's Health. ISSN 1049-3867. https://doi.org/10.1016/j.whi.2004.08.002

Merriam-Webster. (n.d.). Continuum. In Merriam-Webster.com dictionary. Retrieved August 28, 2024, from https://www.merriam-webster.com/dictionary/continuum.

Online Etymology Dictionary. (n.d.) Etymology of continuum by etymonline. https://www.etymonline.com/word/continuum.

Papero, D., Frost, R., Havstad, L., & Noone, R. (2018). Natural systems thinking and the human family. *Systems* 6(2):19. https://doi.org/10.3390/systems6020019

Solnit, R. (2018). *Call them by their true names*. Haymarket Books. ASIN B07C5W7KDC

7 Multiple Continuum Assessment

Given the freedom of the Research Workshop at the Family Center, the idea of juxtaposing multiple continuums simultaneously first occurred to me in 1999 as a way to encompass important aspects of the menopause transition and their interactions. Twenty-five years later with the data in, this type of reckoning still applies.

When I first began working within the medical system as a social worker, I learned the "SOAP" system for clinical notes by which all providers involved with a patient could follow their progress and current status. At that time, the elements were S = subjective (the patient's view of their condition and reason for seeking care); O = objective (results of physical exam and diagnostics performed); A = assessment (summary of patient data, relevant history, major diagnosis, and clinical stability); and P = plan (problem list by level of acuity with plan of action for each). Recently there has been discussion in the context of electronic medical records to change the order to APSO to streamline ongoing care and evaluation. This in turn has been balanced by worry doing such would give less countenance to patient views (Shoolin, 2013).

As a social worker, my base recording was the "psychosocial assessment," described as "a complete comprehensive evaluation of the emotional, mental, and physical health of a person," including "the person's perception of themselves and their ability to function in the community" (socialworkportal.com).

For purposes of the MAPS data, I proposed three continuums: the menopause transition, the relationship system, and resources. The continuums were proposed as both intra- and interrelated, as are the ideas "bio-psycho-social."

The Menopause Transition

There is a reason the menopause transition became known familiarly as "The Change" since this is what is most notable, and sometimes most confounding, to the women going through it, as well as their relationship networks, and their health care providers. While individual experiences vary considerably, the alteration of patterns managed for decades in one's own style and according to one's own circumstances can create challenges. Beginning changes

DOI: 10.4324/9781003540830-9

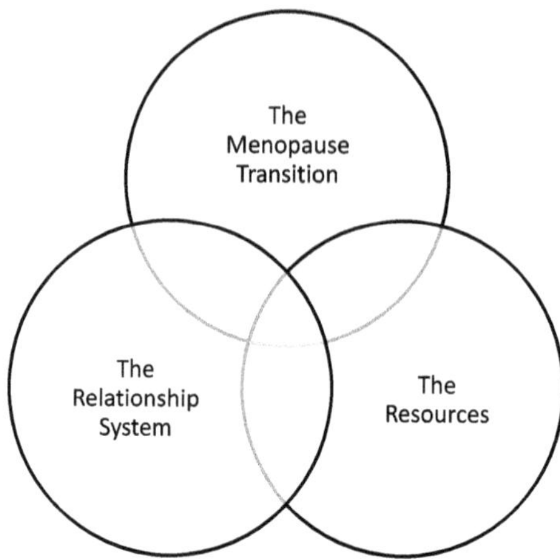

Figure 7.1 Multiple Continuum Assessment Venn Diagram © Nomi Redding reprinted with permission.

The Venn Diagram depicts three overlapping circles representing the mutual influence of multiple variables in the midlife woman's transition to menopause, including The Menopause Transition, The Relationship System, and The Resources available to her. The diagram can also serve as a template for any dynamic process of a living system showing simultaneously its fluidity and continuing interaction of factors.

may seem quite subtle, with women vaguely aware their menses are coming a little earlier or a little later than they expect, that breasts may seem more sore, and that feelings may seem a little more tender and somewhat surprising. Over time, however, it becomes clear: "SOMETHING IS HAPPENING"! Whether "the change" takes center stage in one's life or remains in the periphery relates to the totality of the current situation. For my mom, having heavy periods at the time my father had one serious (and ultimately life-threatening) illness after another, the menopause transition remained in the background. Her diligent routine of regular medical and dental appointments shifted to accompanying my dad to his, making special meals for him, and learning medical procedures from my sister on his behalf. After his death, picking up the pieces of her changed life, she caught up with her own health.

For some women, it may not be the cycles per se which dominate attention, but other physical, emotional, or social symptoms which emerge and require management. Others experience the transition as no big deal. Whatever its nature, arriving at the final menstrual period is often a relief expressed as being "on the other side." Several of the long-term participants referred to the "postmenopausal zest" Margaret Mead described (Quental et al, 2023). Some mentioned "less drama, more satisfaction" in their lives as well as a reconciliation to the aging process. And some, along the way, expressed a certain wistfulness for lost patterns and the potential to reproduce.

Table 7.1 Continuum Categories

CONTINUUM CATEGORIES

The menopause transition

Signs and symptoms		*Level of intervention*	
interesting	troublesome	inexpensive	costly
few	many	less time	more time
mild	intense	easy	difficult

Success of intervention

well satisfied dissatisfied

The relationship system

Quality of support network		*Stability of support network*	
benefit	burden	more secure	less stable

System stress load

low system stress high system stress

Resources

Medical system

beneficial unsatisfactory

Complementary

beneficial unsatisfactory

Self-guided

many few

I note three broad continuums for the menopause transition: (1) signs and symptoms; (2) interventions; and (3) success of interventions (as perceived by the participants), keeping in mind these categories are intertwined in each person's life experience.

Signs and Symptoms

This continuum has several categories, including symptoms from interesting to troublesome, few to many, and mild to intense. Uncertainty dominates the years before the final menstrual period. Whether the inability to predict interferes with life functioning or is simply curious has everything to do with how comforted a person is by the familiar, how much space she has in her daily life to experiment with different ways to manage the new, and the balance in her relationships between beneficial and burdensome.

Most troublesome for participants at perimenopause were heavy, frequent, and painful periods, headaches and/or flashes which interfered with sleep, and family or work situations which could not readily accommodate change. The occasionally experienced cognitive "fog" could be amusing or worrisome. A participant working in a busy office found it embarrassing not to be at the top of her game with details the job demanded, while another described easily adapting to asking people their names. Lost sleep (often linked to night sweats) spilled over to other areas of life, leading to low energy and fatigue. Hot flashes could be funny or embarrassing, intriguing or barely noted. Atypical exaggerations of mood could be scary for women and alarming for family members who might ask, "Are you okay?" And participants having heavy periods paid careful attention to clothing while carrying menstrual products everywhere. With the end to flow, buying new underwear could be a cause for celebration. Each woman drew her own lines for how much she could tolerate with grace and good humor and when it was time to seek help for unrelenting and perplexing issues.

Level of Intervention

At the time participants reached out for assistance, they had an already established history for the resources they considered most reliable and already knew were most available to them. As a group, project participants were readers and listeners, people accustomed to being in charge of their own lives and decisions. Many entered the study with their own hypotheses of what was "off" as well as standards for what options they would consider to address problems.

Categories included in the continuum for intervention are: no expense to considerable cost; minimal to significant time invested; and easy to difficult recovery. While the sample population of the study was relatively homogeneous by many demographic factors, from the beginning I could see variation in how participants had traditionally approached their periods and now anticipated menopause. Some were very aware of their cycles, always kept records, and visited health care providers regularly. Others never kept records and seldom sought professional advice. All had sufficient interest in this stage of menstrual life to join the project, at least at the first interview.

Acute and unmanageable symptoms correlated with the severity of interventions chosen. For women having a miserable time with heavy, frequent and/or painful periods, electing hysterectomy or endometrial ablation seemed useful options, sometimes after having already experienced graduated steps of prescription medications. The scheduling of medical procedures was often influenced by work schedules and insurance coverage, and most participants who opted for them were ready to move on past them with some relief. A few women with heavy periods whose doctors recommended hormone therapy or surgery chose to "wait it out" without treatment. While those without surgical interventions had time to adjust to the reality of no periods, some of the women with hysterectomy who had not had children experienced a time of melancholy regret. On the other hand, those who had never planned to reproduce were relieved to be finished with that possibility.

Finally, there were women who felt their own reproduction was complete and looked forward to the next generation adding to the family. In some instances, the end of the participant's cycles and the birth of her grandchildren coincided.

Success of Intervention

The women whose symptoms represented major stressors disrupting their daily lives reported satisfaction with the interventions they had chosen and by and large, were pleased with the results. Sometimes surgical findings clarified problems they had had, which was both enlightening and validating. Women on conventional Premphase and Prempro regimens had mixed results. More satisfaction was reported with the elimination of periods altogether than treatments which dictated certain on-and-off days and required more intensive management. There were women who adapted prescriptions to fit their own life situations which amounted to conducting their own trial-and-error experiments with varying outcomes.

Participants who selected "natural" hormone options such as creams and troches often reported they couldn't really tell a difference. As a subgroup they tended to go on-and-off these regimens or to use them "when I remember." A couple of women continued to note symptoms of cycling in their data books following hysterectomy without oophorectomy. On average these participants tended to be younger than those without medical interventions. Since a good percentage of the study population remained in the project past their final periods, we were able to see how relatively quickly menstrual life faded to the background ("that's over now") as the focus shifted to other areas of life and aspects of aging.

Success of interventions reported by the participants fully integrated with what was available; reported in recent research; recommended by health care providers; and/or covered by insurance. The controversy over the WHI results created unexpected challenges for both providers and participants as they pivoted from popular regimens toward alternative choices. Then as symptoms waned, some of the women moved away from medications and supplements altogether.

The Relationship System

In their recent article, Papero and colleagues (Papero et al., 2018) wrote:
systems thinking looks at the way in which the parts interact with one another to create the larger whole, and how the larger whole, in turn, regulates the parts which make it up. The back-and-forth interaction between the parts and the whole is observable and predictable in living systems. Systems thinking focuses on the facts of how the parts of a network interact and under what conditions the patterns of interaction change.

In a subsequent article, Papero (2021) elaborated: "Individuals occupy functioning positions or roles in the family system. Each functioning position serves a purpose for the individual and for the system." While Dr. Bowen's original eight theoretical concepts were drawn from his direct observation of and work with families, systems thinking can be applied to other relationship networks, such as work systems, friendships, communities, and nations.

The broad continuums for the relationship systems of the participants include benefit to burden; more secure to less stable; and low to high system stress load. Whether relationships are seen as predominantly beneficial or difficult also speaks to the functional position of the participant in the various systems to which she belongs. Network stability encompasses whether contact is continuing or cut off and its nature. The system stress load can be seen in the acute stressors reported by the women in their annual updates, as well as chronic issues over time.

Benefit/Burden of Support Network

Women at midlife have multiple roles in their families, friendships, and communities. Some participants found their partners interested and willing to journey with them through the territory of changing bodies, goals, and markers of aging. Other primary relationships could not ford this passage easily, sometimes ending, and sometimes enduring rocky periods which ultimately resolved. A key sticking point was differing expectations. It is characteristic of relationship systems that a change in one person in a relationship requires adaptation by others, particularly if the person making the shift is central to the group. Participants reported their partners' reactions to symptoms the women were experiencing, and conversely their own reactions to changes in the partner's life and health. Launching children and planning for retirement could be key areas where viewpoints diverged, which might leave each person feeling upset and lonely. At the other end of this continuum, a number of participants referred to their reinvigorated relationships, with children raised, more time for each other, and shared or developing interests.

On the family diagrams, we charted births, educational milestones, marriages and divorces of children, and births of grandchildren. The women's multigenerational families were also changing as their menstrual cycles advanced to completion. Sometimes the demands of children, elders, and partners outweighed caring for one's own health. On the other hand, women found it could be calming and joyful to experience happy events and turning points with those closest to them. And sometimes there was a type of balance in that while one generation was a stressor another could serve as a resource to help.

All participants were daughters and the health and aging of their parents impacted their lives in specific ways. Women could be called to serve their original families as they had traditionally or needing to learn new skills or adapt relationships to meet the changing circumstances. It was particularly challenging if the needs of dependent children, older parents, and partners overlapped, requiring nimble, and sometimes exhausting, compensations on the part of the participants. Parents contributed both positive and negative examples for the women as they approached their own later years. Mothers, sisters, and other female relatives sometimes proved invaluable resources offering advice, comfort, or at least a listening ear.

Alterations in family structure could be anticipated and unexpected at the same time. The women who most comfortably "rode the waves" seemed to have space to breathe and think, support from their relationships, and the option to approach the transition with more interest than urgency.

Stability of Relationship Network

Factors which impacted the stability of participants' relationship networks include: the sheer number of changes experienced (particularly in a short amount of time); whether those changes were anticipated or took them by surprise; and whether the changes were welcome or painful. Typically, death and divorce rattled the women much more than, for instance, the planned-for high school graduations of their children. For some shifts, one could conjure a bell curve experience similar to the trip through the menopause transition itself: from subtle or expected changes to energy-demanding crisis points to ease into the next era. This contrasted with experiences for which there was no preparation accompanied by an abrupt sense of dislocation.

The category of continuity to discontinuity was readily visible updating participant diagrams as well as by verbal report in our annual interviews. When the family system or friendship base or community adds or loses members, adjustment is required from everyone who remains. How preoccupying this becomes is a function of the structure of the system: are these central people much relied on or peripherally present? How much energy is available to deal effectively with discontinuous times and when are they most likely to be destabilizing, at least for a time? Negotiating discontinuous events with flexibility and presence could benefit all.

Emotional cutoff within Bowen Theory is described as a naturally occurring process in all families to greater and lesser degrees Bowen (1978). It is most exaggerated in relationships which become estranged. During the project years, participants sometimes experienced a period of marked distance from their young adult children. As mothers, it could be particularly challenging to allow breathing room for the child to initiate reconciliation, while also attending to one's own life and keeping the door open to the other generation. Another area of notable cutoff sometimes occurred at times of a significant death in the family, for instance between siblings attempting to process possessions as well as emotions or between adult stepchildren and their parents' surviving partners. There could also be times of tension between siblings as their elderly parents became ill and needed care. Who was going to do what for how long was an ongoing negotiation, not only with brothers and sisters but with participants' spouses and children as well.

Cutoff in its most subtle form can manifest even in families who live next door to each other but never share innermost thoughts and feelings, instead tiptoeing around sensitive issues. It is one thing for people to know who they can depend on to take them to the hospital in an emergency, it is quite another to experience the comfort of a nonjudgmental and thoughtful listener. Participants typically knew whom they could trust to share confidences and offer useful advice.

System Stress Load

When I was in clinical practice I used to refer to "crunch times" with my clients, when their family diagrams would "light up" with happenings in nearly all sectors: births, deaths, marriages, divorces, moves, job changes, arrests, hospitalizations. Change brings uncertainty and requires adaptation to new circumstances. Whether positive or negative, people note the drain and strain on their brains. After the stillbirth of our first child, events in the world "out there" felt very far away, my brain fogged, my heart heavy. After the full-term birth of our second daughter, I noted very similar effects on functioning although the affect was opposite. The big event was needing to buy diapers because we had run out, whereas the fact President Reagan had been shot seemed quite far away.

For women in the study, when major shifts in relationships coincided with significant symptoms in menstrual life, choices about management were heavily influenced by system demands. For those whose functioning was relied on by important others, participants might decide to either ignore their own problems in the hope they would go away or, oppositely, opt for quick and serious interventions to "get over it." Those who traditionally were the most symptomatic family members might have a tougher time than usual, requiring even more care from family members or friends. Or, they could step up to function until the crisis was over and the system established its usual balance. This balance included the needs of the extended family as well as the people in one's own home.

Resources

Participants entered the project with their own histories and expectations of medical resources: their doctors or alternative health care practitioners, their pharmacists, and health food advisors. The chief category for this continuum is to what degree the women found their resources to be useful to them. The medical system included physicians, certified nurse practitioners, hospitals and clinics, pharmacists, and prescription medications. Complementary resources included mind-body therapies, body-based practices, and over-the-counter supplements, as well as energy work and naturopathic medicine. I reserved the category of "self-guided" resources to include reading and record-keeping, self-observation, and self-care. The participants in this study for the most part chose an "all of the above" approach, relying on practitioners in both conventional and complementary medicine, some prescription medications and some over-the-counter supplements as well as compounded hormone treatments, body work, exercise, their own research through self-study and news reports. This was a well-educated group accustomed to making informed choices.

Medical System

Tracking with the women the medical system resources in the perimenopausal era seemed reminiscent of having gathered their medical histories at baseline. Recommendations were heavily influenced by new studies, the culture in which they lived, and the era. For the participants who enrolled in the older age groups, there was a decided emphasis on hormone therapy, not so much "if" but "when" and "which?" Women who took the stand they were not interested in treating a "natural process" could find themselves "swimming against the tide." Some changed doctors to find a professional more in tune with their personal philosophy. There were women who had few symptoms requiring treatment; if they were people who had always had regular annual physical examinations, they generally continued in this pattern and reported findings of lab values and other tests. There was another group of participants who only made medical appointments if they were needing help for specific conditions.

Women with the most problematic periods went through a time in which they might be making many more medical appointments than usual sometimes with multiple practitioners who occasionally gave conflicting opinions. This was an additional stress for participants: time-consuming, expensive, and disheartening. Other participants were quite appreciative of receiving treatment in a straightforward manner that resolved their problems. Pharmacists and nurse practitioners within doctor's offices were often regarded as quite valuable resources in the problem-solving process and sometimes viewed as people with more time to discuss and explain than the physicians.

Complementary

Depending on where they lived and their own preferences many women found a bevy of complementary practitioners available and received a variety of services offered, including chiropractic, acupuncture, massage, structural integration, and yoga classes. To some extent participants reported that the atmosphere in these offices seemed more relaxed and spacious than the general medical practices. They valued being heard and recognized as a whole person with a life bigger than the menopause transition. However, without insurance reimbursement, there could be trade-offs in which type of help to seek.

I include the friendship network as part of this category, as participants could find their female friends and some family members extremely useful as resources with whom to share experiences, gather information, and feel less alone during major changes. There could be cross-fertilization with informal resources being the source for seeking professional and other complementary resources. This was not necessarily a two-way proposition; in that it was much more likely a woman would express she was seeing a certain doctor or taking a certain supplement on recommendation from her close friend than that the doctor or pharmacist would question the participant as to who she had at home and in her life as a source of support.

Self-guided

Regardless of who was consulted, participants ultimately realized they were in charge of their own decisions. To that end, they often mentioned books they had read, articles they had seen, and podcasts they had listened to which caused them to think further or differently about what they were experiencing, and sometimes reinforced it. Listening to the women, I realized they were running their own research experiments with hypotheses about what caused and what helped certain bodily changes and symptoms. They could make adjustments accordingly, based on their own observations. Some sifted through professional advice in terms of what they agreed with and what they didn't. From the first year on, a number of participants commented how useful record keeping was in their lives, for noting changes, anticipating differences, and communicating with their health care providers around actual data.

Managing Health at Midlife

It's a good plan to avoid spring allergies by leaving the state. I am looking forward to getting a hearing aid in the next few months. I have set a goal to walk 12 miles a week.

Being physically active is a lot more work. I am slower and it takes longer to build up my muscle strength and lung capacity. I ache more and I am tired more. Cataracts are growing.

Stress gives me headaches a lot. Anxiety, a lot of times feel too many things going on. Try to compartmentalize. Some days I feel so tired from all the mental, emotional, and physical stuff going on. Older, more creaks, shoulder and back hurt a little bit. Should do yoga and aerobics. Need to lose some weight. Like to eat my chocolate. On my own during the day, don't eat that great.

I think about quitting smoking all the time but it's a difficult step for me to take.

Throughout life I have barged ahead with all kinds of physical activities. It would be nice if I do have cramps or diarrhea not to have to do things. In modern society we barge right ahead.

I don't like the idea that a woman's moods are blamed on her cycle. I hadn't ever noticed that pattern. It's a time for me to give myself space to remove. Native American custom for the woman to remove time for meditation during menstruation.

Didn't think of as a hot flash until quite a bit later, when I read a magazine. Get warm all at once-take sweater off, cool off. Now just warm, not sweaty. Difference in lean body mass is not true weight gain. Distribution of weight is different – more on stomach, breasts have changed with self-exam, more mushy. Aging? Hormonal changes? Don't think there's the same strength in your body. Skin texture is different in face. Basically, I have been very healthy. More wrinkles, gray hair. Read the article where hand strength decreases with hormonal changes. Notice with taking lid off using garden clippers. Have to work harder in a small area to accomplish same thing. Probably shouldn't have read the article.

References

Bowen, M. (1978). Theory in the practice of psychotherapy. *Family Therapy in Clinical Practice.* New York: Jason Aronson. Reprinted from *Family Therapy* (1976). Ed. Guerin, P. New York: Gardner Press.

Papero, D.V. (2020). Developing a systems model for family assessment. In M.N. Keller, & R.J. Noone (Eds.) *Handbook of Bowen family systems theory and research methods: A systems model for family research.* New York and Abington: Routledge. ISBN: 978-1-138-47812-1.

Papero, D.V. (2021). Murray Bowen's contribution to the study of complex human systems. *Family Systems* 16(1):43–67.

Papero, D., Frost, R., Havstad, L., & Noone, R. (2018). Natural systems thinking and the human family. *Systems* 6(2):19. https://doi.org/10.3390/systems6020019

Quental, C., Gaviria, P., & del Bucchia, C. (2023). The dialectic of (menopause) zest: Breaking the mold of organizational irrelevance. *Gender Work Organ* 30:1816–1838. Wileyonlinelibrary.com/journal/gwao https://doi.org/10.1111/gwao.13017

Shoolin, J., Ozeran, L., Hamann, C., & Bria, W. II. (2013). Association of medical directors information systems consensus on inpatient electronic health record documentation. *Applied Clinical Informatics* 4:293–303. https://doi.org:10.4338/ACI-2013-02-R-0012

Sindhu, K. (2020). *What are SOAP notes?* https://www.wolterskluwer.com/en/expert-insights/what-are-soap-notes

8 What Helps?

The Fundamental Nature of Communication

Naturalist David Attenborough ended his Attenborough (1979) BBC documentary series "Life on Earth" with Episode 13: "The Compulsive Communicators." The phrase stayed with me as I worked with clients, interviewed participants, and lived my life. Communication was foundational to my profession, and has been indispensable to this research. Further, good communication has everything to do with a tolerable progression through the menopause transition whereas garbled or problematic communication may create extra stress. Numerous studies of aging have confirmed that a key to life satisfaction, good health, and longevity is meaningful relationships (Busse & Maddox, 1986). This aspect outdistances advances of modern medicine in predicting beneficial outcomes (Novotney, 2011).

At base, communication is defined as information exchanged through a common system of symbols, signs, or behavior. Communication as a field encompasses not only the qualities of the exchange but also the tools which are employed. As one example, in my mother's nearly century-long lifetime, the world "shrank" while modes of communication multiplied: from the radio by which her family listened to the fireside chats of FDR, to the first televisions of my own childhood and my daughter's first computer, to the internet by which Mom then kept in touch with her grandchildren from a geographic distance. Phones went from party lines with simple call letters or digits (and cords!) to cellular wireless service all over the world. To Mom's credit she stayed current through the decades and was one of the few residents in her assisted living facility to use Facebook.

What follows is a discussion of the topic of communication through categories with particular relevance to the research project. They include: the multigenerational family and other relationship networks; deep listening and the cultivation of one's own voice; the wide-ranging effects of compassion; and the importance of collaboration.

DOI: 10.4324/9781003540830-10

The Multigenerational Family and Other Relationship Networks

Bowen Theory centrally reminds that any given individual is embedded in a complex system arrangement of biological and acquired family members through generations as well as important others in the present. The family diagram constructed at enrollment and updated each year for all continuing participants in the MAPS study underlined that each woman was not on a solitary journey through the menopause transition but moving through multiple networks of ongoing relationships. The diagram served as a visual prompt which could lessen the intensity of the present moment or at least invite a broader context through which symptoms or stressors could be understood and thought through. In the "crunch times," people could feel less "crazy" and more thoughtful about what was actually under their control and what wasn't.

Project participants could easily point to their most troublesome relationships and the challenge it was to manage them along with the changes in their own bodies, as well as to express gratitude when receiving support and useful information. There was variation between the participants in terms of the number and quality of functional relationships available to them and how well those ties fit (or didn't) with their own view of self, which in turn could also be evolving. What could be less clear to the women was how their own automatic reactions to current events might have originated in past generations, particularly if there were gaps in historical knowledge or "static on the line" in the present. Andrea Schara (2015) has written, "Each of us probably 'inherits' a position in our family depending on the family's history, its current needs and our natural abilities. There is a tendency to function according to one's position in the group." At the same time, one's functional position can vary according to the particular group at hand. I remember even as a child taking note of the difference in my great aunt who never married and lived with members of her extended family all of her life when she was at work and when she was at home. During the day, she functioned as an extremely competent executive secretary in a large corporation. When she came home, to my ears she sounded like the younger sister to her older brother and seemed, in so far as I could tell, to be content to have his wife, her sister-in-law, manage the household.

The study was constructed to focus year after year on the participants' partners, children (if any), parents, siblings (if any), and extended family members. In addition, the women frequently volunteered information about their friendships, work systems, and involvements in community and religious organizations (Pivodic et al 2024 and Shah 2024). Through what was known and not known, said and not said, and present or absent in the diagram as well as the personal interviews, a picture emerged over time for each person of how connected or disconnected to others she felt and to what extent that impacted her perimenopausal passage. Especially disruptive were situations in which a previously supportive relationship disappeared or came into question. Conversely, it was quite comforting for people in one's network to step up in unexpected ways to remove burdens or barriers.

Deep Listening and The Cultivation of One's Own Voice

In his version of the five basic precepts common to all Buddhist traditions, Thich Nhat Hanh (1998) included "loving speech and deep listening" as the Fourth Mindfulness Training. The practice includes giving each person respectful opportunity to be genuinely heard without interruption or correction and in turn each speaking in a way that can be readily heard by others. Practitioners note how helpful (and how rare in modern society) deep listening is. This truth fits nicely with my experience in clinical work as well. The greatest compliment a client could pay was, "You really listened to me." The participants in the research study expressed the same benefit: being heard without judgment.

Surgeon and writer Atul Gawande (2002) has shared Cassell (1991) perspective that patients who receive a measure of understanding can experience reduced stress, apart from any medical treatments. This is a two-way street when patients are given respectful space to develop and express their own voices.

The MAPS population by and large consisted of women who were accustomed to speaking their minds and assuming they would have choices. I think of participants who spoke in terms of interviewing doctors to see who might be most helpful to their concerns and made a distinction between hiring the physician to consult while retaining the responsibility for decision-making for themselves.

Sometimes it was easier for the women to access and express a well-defined voice "out in the world" as opposed to dealing with intimate others. The reverse was also true, for women who felt in command in their own homes but could be intimidated to speak with someone "in authority." There is no "one size fits all" approach to the most comforting way in which to share problems or to receive help, but across the board the sense of being understood was welcome.

An additional dimension of communication is the category beyond words: the so-called "nonverbal communication" of body language, facial expressions, tone, and pauses in speech. Family members in particular are quite sensitive to the lack of match between what is being said or heard, seen, and felt. As we grow and age, our modes of communication may also change. I learned first with my father and later with my husband, that what I interpreted as a frown of displeasure could actually signify difficulty hearing. A common experience is sensing someone we love seems upset but receiving a "fine" answer if we ask, "How are you?" Depending on the relationship and the circumstances, sometimes it can lead to a clarifying conversation to simply reflect, "You're hard to believe."

At base, the person with whom we need to be most clear lies within our own skin, as we hear ourselves saying things because we believe it's what the receiver wants to hear, not what we actually think or feel. For participants who decided to redirect their life course, painful conversations followed about what was no longer working for them. At one end of the continuum this could end in a relationship break, and at the other, a refreshed, renewal of the bond with greater freedom available in the older years.

Managing Relationships at Midlife

I'm exceedingly healthy – cholesterol low, blood pressure low, can hike a pretty good distance, not fast. If I had a few more hours sleep, and less mother care, it would be great. Where life is at.

I quit having periods for several months now. I think early but I have two aunts who had menopause in their early 40s. I am thrilled. I took a camping trip by myself – a vacation for the first time in my life no one to talk to from noon Saturday to 4:00 Monday. Loved it, cried when I had to come back.

First time in 23 years of married life my husband knows when my period will be.

No mental disorder-mental symptoms. Assume I retain water, sort of like having the flu, but can't stop what you're doing. My disposition is changed, don't feel well, not in a very good mood. By the start, symptoms are less severe. Feel so sorry for my husband-part of a recurring cycle. Interrupts his emotional and sexual involvement. I am trying to get him to understand it's chronic. He jokes. "Leave me alone" comes as a surprise.

My mother never said a word about this. It's a myth that women just fall apart.

My sexual desire has diminished – it's a challenge on a lot of levels. You feel you have to work at it in a different way. Still in the process.

I feel I have moved into the "old crone," postmenopausal status in my family and society that I have read about. I have less energy, so there's a number of foolish things I absolutely will not put up with. I'm sure from the outside it seems curmudgeonly but from the inside it's "been there, done that. Never again."

The idea of being alone scares me to death. The idea of sharing my life with someone scares me to death. Time keeps marching on.

My life is scheduled around taking care of husband, dad, mother, an old dog, two horses, the house, the yard, cooking, and laundry.

I'm not as obsessed as when I didn't feel good. Really helping me to have a friend going through it, too.

> There are times I think my thinking isn't real clear, especially with
> regard to my job and the tasks assigned. Need to improve lifestyle – I
> don't want to end up like my mom.

The Wide-ranging Effects of Compassion

A natural outcome of deep listening is compassion, which can be expressed ver-
bally and nonverbally. Compassion is action-oriented and emotion-based. Among
many definitions and examples, there is this: "feeling with." Among emotion
researchers, compassion is defined as the feeling that arises when you are con-
fronted with another's suffering and feel motivated to relieve that suffering.

Compassion is relevant to the menopause transition in our relationships
with others, including family and friends, health care providers, and ourselves
(self-compassion). Simply being heard is a good start, and sometimes that
sums up the only interaction needed at the time. I am sensitive to the differences between compassion and "pity" which is not so much feeling with the
other as separate from them. That is quite different than witnessing the "uni-
versality of human suffering." Gawande (2002) cites Carl Schneider (1998), a
professor of law and medicine, who finds that "what patients want most from
doctors isn't autonomy per se; it's competence and kindness."

At the same time, part of the development of one's own voice is acti-
vating care for self. A pervasive finding of the research literature is that
self-compassion leads to authenticity (Neff 2021). To the extent we aren't
dependent on the approval of others for our self-worth, we are freer to express
our true selves. A good technique in communication which enhances listening well while offering genuine interest and care is taking time to pause. We
don't assume that every question requires an immediate answer or that every
situation requires a suggestion. By allowing the space to be thoughtful, we
afford the other person the same opportunity. Good teamwork emerges not
from rushing, but being present in the moment to generate resourcefulness in
the most creative way.

The Importance of Collaboration

Being partnered in a transition can be a great help to weather the changes with
grace and solid decision-making. For the participants, this included loved ones
and friends, health care providers, and all the resources that helped demystify
the process and made them feel accepted. Sharing mutuality of purpose, people
may come to a collaborative process with different perspectives, yet headed
toward the same goal. Participants sometimes changed doctors and marital partners when they felt they weren't being supported in their current reality.

At the other end of the continuum, sometimes the women were gratified to find perfect strangers could be helpful as well as family members, sometimes in surprising ways. The difficulty was when, for instance, there was no break or understanding from spouses, children, or employers on a day that followed lost sleep from night sweats. While participants were trying to catch up with themselves in terms of changes in physical and cognitive functioning, if the expectations of others remained the same, this could stymie collaboration.

Participants shared that they wanted their experiences to be respected and light shed on what accounted for them without being "talked down to" or worse, "tuned out." Where multiple providers were involved, it was confusing and disheartening to have professionals contradicting each other without acknowledging the complexity of the situation. Conversely, it was rewarding and stress-reducing to feel that there was a team operating on one's behalf, with one's own voice counted. A team can accommodate and benefit from a diversity of perspectives if the ultimate goal is well-defined, all input is acknowledged, and there is clear agreement about who has the final say.

References

Attenborough, D. (1979). *Life on earth*. BBC Natural History Documentary Series. Episode 13: The Compulsive Communicators.

Busse, E.W. & Maddox, G.L. (1986). *The Duke Longitudinal Studies of normal aging 1955–1980: Overview of history, design, and findings*. New York: Springer Pub Co. ISBN-13: 978-0826141507.

Cassell, E. (1991). *The nature of suffering and the goals of* medicine. New York: Oxford University Press. ISBN-13: 978-0195089127.

Gawande, A. (2002). *Complications: A surgeon's note on an imperfect science*. New York: Picador Henry Holt and Company. ISBN-13: 978-0312421700.

Nhat Hanh, T. (1998). *The heart of the Buddha's teaching: Transforming suffering into peace, joy, and liberation*. New York: Broadway Books. ISBN-13: 978-0767903691.

Neff, K. (2021). *Fierce self-compassion: How women can harness kindness to speak up, claim their power, and thrive*. New York: Harper. ISBN-13: 978-0062991065.

Novotney, A. (2011). The real secrets to a longer life: Howard S. Friedman says that eating vegetables and going to the gym are not as important to our long-term health as having a rich, proactive life. *American Psychological Association* 42(11). https://www.apa.org/monitor/2011/12/longer-life?fbclid=IwAR2cekd-Gu0xv0qqZqs_Gr5bgYQF5clwfvCnc3iyioWDNi97iLnh2oHOCO

Pivodic, L., van den Block, L., & Pivodic, F. (2024). *Social connection and end-of-life outcomes among older people in 19 countries: A population-based longitudinal study*. Vol. 5. www.thelancet.com/healthy-longevity

Schara, A.M. (2015). Navigating in social systems: Interactions around illness and death. *Family Systems Forum* Fall 2015. Houston: Center for the Study of Natural Systems and the Family.

Schneider, C. (1998). *The practice of autonomy*. New York: Oxford University Press.

Shah, A. (2024). A surprising key to healthy aging: Strong social connections. *Mayo Clinic Press Healthy Aging*. https://mcpress.mayoclinic.org/healthy-aging/

Zaharias, G. (2018). What is narrative-based medicine? *Canadian Family Physician* 64

9 Engaging Complex Living Systems

After reviewing the literature and deciding on a structure for the 2-year pilot project, I named it MAPS, thinking that what we could learn from the study could create elements for a road map useful to midlife women now and in the future. I also liked the acronym because it was easy to remember, so assigned descriptive meanings to each "letter": <u>M</u>enopausal <u>A</u>daptation <u>P</u>rocess <u>S</u>tudy. At the time I had no idea it would grow to a 20-year longitudinal work and how appropriate those terms would prove to be. Enrolling women 34–55 covered "menopausal" pretty well, in terms of pre-, peri, and post. It was natural to think of "adaptation" because I'd never known of a transition that didn't require it, and therefore automatically constituted a "process." There was also never a question that family systems theory would be a basic building block for the project, steeped as I was in the idea (and experience) of lived lives in the context of relationships.

Complex living systems are often described in terms of flow, emergence, multilayered interactions, and dynamic relationships. A woman in menopause transition is part and parcel of many complex living systems: her own body, her family, and the resource network with whom she interacts.

> ### Retirement and Establishing New Priorities
>
> I have never in my life done so little and had it matter so little to me. Amazed at how little I think about work. I had a wonderful send-off this fall. I saw how much difference I've made.
>
> My whole body is different when I don't go to work every day.
>
> I'm heavier. This first year of retirement is my freshman year. I've lived large (+20#). Still comparatively reduced libido, but my husband and I have our own loving rhythm. I am so content 86% of the time. I garden and walk my dog and read and cook. I'm being a good neighbor for the first time.

DOI: 10.4324/9781003540830-11

I'm really very happy. I feel peaceful, calm with myself. I am trying to hang on another 2½ years with the company ahead of retirement. I've done some serious looking into finishing my degree.

I have stepped down out of supervision. It has taken me this past year to feel this job is under control and having a good pace at work. Tremendously contented right now and excited about school. I have watched both parents retire and become couch potatoes – not going to do that.

Since not working, I can regulate room temperature and have fewer hot flashes.

Now I have my children basically grown, I have more time, to volunteer, meditate. I love not being pressured. I really do enjoy having the house to myself and wouldn't want to go back to having young children. I do feel more empowered in my womanhood, taking belly dancing. I can be more self-reflective.

I turned 50, didn't realize it would be that much of a landmark. It started me thinking about what I want to do for the rest of my life which is kind of neat. I am rediscovering things I've had in my past I like and didn't have time to keep up with before. I'm trying to find a way to re-integrate.

Complicated versus Complex

While human lives can certainly become complicated, complexity introduces other levels of reality to consider which offer both challenge and opportunity. In *Getting to Maybe: How the World Is Changed*, Westley et al. (2007) depict differences in simple, complicated, and complex problems. They write: "In complex situations there are no final answers," and advocate a mindset "framed by inquiry not certitude, one that embraces paradoxes and tolerates multiple perspectives."

It can be the case that certain prescriptions for one midlife woman do not work similarly for another, or for the same woman from one time to another. While the media tends to distil multilayered research reports into "sound bites" and pharmaceutical companies feel pressured to market potentially promising drugs in the short term without foreknowledge of what may be coming down the road, the midlife woman needs all the wisdom she has gained from her own lived life and history to make decisions in uncertain environments.

A truth increasingly recognized and researched is that dichotomies are easy to fall into, hard to climb out of, and invariably fall short of explanatory power. One of the editors of *Rethinking Cancer*, Marta Bertolaso, presented in her earlier book *Philosophy of Cancer: A Dynamic and Relational View*

(2016) that it was not necessary to opt for either reductionist or holistic perspectives, but to include learning from both to arrive at the most useful solutions for complex dilemmas. Similarly, Sandra Mitchell in *Unsimple Truths: Science, Complexity, and Policy* (2009, 2012), argued:

> there is a mismatch between the current sciences of complex behaviors and standard philosophical criteria for scientific knowledge … To begin to understand many aspects of our complex world … we need to expand our conceptual frameworks to accommodate contingency, dynamic robustness, and deep uncertainty.

Victoria Team (2021), a senior research fellow in the School of Nursing and Midwifery at Monash University and health services research fellow at Monash Partners, concluded in her chapter "Perimenopause: The Body, Mind, and Spirit in Transition" in *Musings on Perimenopause and Menopause*:

> My other suggestion is to avoid dichotomizing perimenopausal attitudes and experiences as either positive or negative. Taking into account all aspects of women's lives-including the various social, cultural, psychological, and hormonal factors that may shape them-and given that this transition occurs over a lengthy period of time, women can expect to experience both positive and negative changes in different stages of perimenopause.

Menopause can present problems to be solved and challenges to daily living at the same time it is a predictable and accepted natural fact of life. The best help recognizes the variation not just from woman to woman but from one time to another in a given woman's life, one embedded in a web of her relationships and changing circumstances. By recognizing and respecting the complexity of the process, we can better understand and assist each person's transition.

Levels of Focus, Variation, and Uncertainty

In *The Systems View of Life: A Unifying Vision*, co-authors Capra and Luisi (2014) identified seven characteristics of systems thinking: (1) shift of perspective from the parts to the whole; (2) inherent multidisciplinarity; (3) from objects to relationships; (4) from measuring to mapping; (5) from quantities to qualities; (6) from structures to processes; and (7) from objective to epistemic science. In *Period*, Clancy (2023) echoes the points of systems thinking "… if we truly want to understand menstruation it's better to seek to understand processes rather than outcomes and to explore variation rather than dichotomize people as normal or pathological." And Dr. Treloar (1967) in the article which jump-started my quest to learn more by talking to real women, "Variation of the Human Menstrual Cycle through Reproductive Life" foreshadowed Clancy: "Variation is the rule … All menstrual histories show individualities that make the norms provided by statistical procedures useful only for comparisons of groups of persons."

With the idea not to discard every aspect of reductionist techniques, but to put them in perspective of the whole experience, the central task is to be clear on which level one is focusing without losing sight of the context. One measure of FSH will not determine a woman is "in menopause" and therefore, should do the protocol du jour of the moment. It can, however, represent a glimpse that something is happening. Equally as, and sometimes more important, is the woman's own observations and internal sense as well as her tolerance for living with fluctuations. To the extent any person, or any given line of inquiry, or management group, can engage uncertainty, the opportunity exists for the emergence (recognition) of new paradigms for understanding the richness inherent in complex systems.

In a white paper "Complexity Science in Health Care: Aspirations, Approaches, Applications and Accomplishments", Braithwaite et al (2017) summarize:

> Complexity science is not a new idea, but in 2017 its time has surely come in relation to health care provision. Health systems around the world are struggling with the unprecedented interacting challenge of-among others-increased life expectancy (and the concomitant increase in chronic illness, multi-morbidity and frailty), technological progress (both real and imagined), the convergence of "health" and "care" needs (along with increasing, messy disputes over who should pay for them), fragmentation of services, mismatches between work force supply and system demand, mushrooming of regulations and protocols, diminishing public trust in health professionals, and shrinking budgets. On top of that, a suite of actions in the area of preventive public policy could reduce the burden of disease, if only governments felt able to tackle vested interests that perpetuate poor health.

Building Bridges

Given the endless well of challenge complexity presents, it requires us not to take on projects as the "Lone Ranger," but in concert with others, humbly, and respectfully. Commenting on "intellectual humility," Ravi Chandra writing in the Greater Good newsletter from Berkeley cites a study in the *Journal of Personality Assessment* (2023) which proposed "two key dimensions of intellectual humility: self-directed vs. other-directed and internal vs. expressed. Internal and self-directed humility "requires … questioning yourself and your assumptions," whereas internal and other-directed humility "requires asking yourself whether you can understand and relate to others' beliefs and perspectives." Expressed and other-directed intellectual humility "requires relating to others in good faith." I think of Thich Nhat Hanh's suggestions: to self "Are you sure?" and to the other, "You are partially correct."

Working in the hospital as a young medical social worker, I found it remarkable the immediate caring relationships formed by families waiting in ICU and ER waiting rooms regardless of their demographics in the outside world. This is consistent with key bases of our humanity: to relate to, empathize with, and reach out to others. Women participating in online chats or with friends in person experience considerable relief that they "are not alone" when transacting confusing transitions. In addition, evaluations of medical personnel (as well as staff morale) increase with a sense of connection between patient and provider. Vaill (1996) commented on this human element of learning, the qualities of which he references as "moral philosophy": "honesty about self, starting from ignorance (not knowing in order to find fresh questions), action (not just thought) imperative for learning, in a spirit of friendship, for the purpose of doing good in the world."

In her book *Real Life*, meditation teacher Sharon Salzberg (2023) stated: Caregiving is a distinctive kind of role in that it literally requires the practice of compassion, opening one's heart, on the job. Caregiving is often a complex endeavor, replete with joys and sorrows, an incredible opening of the heart coupled with the bitter after taste of feeling we are never able to do enough. Along that continuum, being able to share with colleagues and receive support at home from friends and family, is essential to moderating the highs and lows of service, and rising to greet another day.

Slowing Down to Better Represent

In July of 2023, the Society for Menstrual Cycle Research held its 24th Biennial Conference in Bethesda, Maryland. The overall conference theme was "The Period Is Political: Menstrual Research, Policy, and Practice." I was honored to have the opportunity to present a Flash Talk I titled, "Slowing Down to Better Represent: The Role of Longitudinal Studies in Menopause Research," based on the 20-year MAPS project. I said,

> I have learned longitudinal studies are a gift to researchers and participants alike: to be able to be present with lived lives over time and in context is rich and varied, and puts us in touch with the rhythm and flow (if you will) of nature as it unfolds. As we represent the process in its complexity, we are present listeners and recorders of the process.

My first slides depicted the process as multiple continuums, each influencing and being influenced by the others, which is entirely consistent with the models of my mentors, and the ever-growing field of complexity in natural systems. In retrospect, I was lucky indeed to happen in 1989 on a research topic which naturally lent itself to longitudinal study, to be supported by colleagues doing similar investigations, and to launch into a subject of concern to diligent and curious women. Having finished this particular journey, I am more than ever convinced of the worthiness of study over time and in context, and am heartened to see current writing from a number of fields echoing this idea even as the world continues to challenge at nearly the speed of light with hardly a moment to breathe, let alone ponder, and simply let development unfold.

References

Bertolaso, M. (2016). *Philosophy of cancer: A dynamic and relational view*. Springer Science and Business Media. https://doi.org/10.1007/978-94-024-0865-2

Braithwaite, J., Churruca, K., Ellis, L.A., & Long, J.C. (2017). *Complexity science in healthcare: Aspirations, approach, applications & accomplishments: A White Paper*. Centre for Healthcare Resilience & Implementation Science (CHRIS). Australia Institute of Health Innovation (AIHI). https://www.researchgate.net/publication/319643112

Capra, F., & Luisi, P. (2014). *The systems view of life: A unifying vision*. Cambridge University Press. ISBN: 978-13166116437.

Chandra, R. (2023). The eight kinds of humility that can help you stay grounded. https://greatergood.berkeley.edu.

Clancy, K. (2023). *Period: The real story of menstruation*. Princeton University Press. ISBN-13: 978-0691191317.

Mitchell, S. (2009, 2012). *Unsimple truths: Science, complexity, and policy*. University of Chicago Press. ISBN-13: 978-0226006628.

Salzberg, S. (2023). *Real life: The journey from isolation to openness and freedom*. Flatiron Books. ISBN-13: 07-9781250835739

Team, V. (2021). Perimenopause: The body, mind and spirit in transition. In Dillaway and Wershler (Eds.) (2020). *Musings on perimenopause and menopause: Identity, experience, transition*. Bradford, Ontario, Canada: Demeter Press. ISBN-13: 978-1772582857.

Treloar, A.E., Boynton, R.E., Behn, B.G., & Brown, B.W. (1967). Variation of the human menstrual cycle through reproductive life. *International Journal of Fertility* 12(1 Pt 2):77–126.

Vaill, P. (1996). *Learning as a way of being: Strategies for survival in a world of permanent white water*. San Francisco, CA: Jossey-Bass, Inc. ISBN-13: 978-0787902469.

Westley, F., Zimmerman, B., & Patton, M. (2007). *Getting to maybe: How the world is changed*. Toronto: Vintage Canada, a division of Random House of Canada. ISBN-13: 978-0679314448.

Part 3
Conclusions and Recommendations

Dealing with uncertainty challenges medical providers and researchers to attend effectively to patient views; at the same time, it calls on those asking for help to be clear about their expectations and concerns. What follows are observations and suggestions for those in the three key roles: transitioning persons and those closest to them; health services providers; and researchers in the menopause transition as well as other living systems.

DOI: 10.4324/9781003540830-12

10 For Women and Those Who Love Them

Right Health

Buddhist traditions speak of the Noble Eightfold Path as the route to engaging and transforming suffering. Each of the eight begins with the word "Right" which is also meant as "skillful" or "wholesome" in contrast to "wrong," "not yet skillful," or "unwholesome." Jerome Freedman (2014) is a mindfulness meditation teacher and a cancer survivor since 1997. A long-time practitioner in the Plum Village tradition of Zen Master Thich Nhat Hanh (2006) and a certified teacher of the Enneagram, he has identified seven strategies that have helped him to survive:

- Be your own advocate
- Investigate alternatives
- Make health-promoting lifestyle changes
- Practice daily meditation
- Create your own medical team
- Reach out to others
- Give back

I suggest that each person can design for herself her own elements of "Right Health." Wherever we start from, and whatever our current circumstances and past history, it is up to us to define for ourselves what makes life worth living. Evidence from a number of studies and perspectives shows that whatever their personal definitions, people who have time and space to consider options, the freedom to put them into action, as well as important others in their relationship networks generally report more life satisfaction and enjoy healthier outcomes than those who don't share those same advantages.

Self-Care

Midlife women have a decided tendency to put wishes, wants, or goals for themselves at the bottom of their "to-do" lists, following those of family

DOI: 10.4324/9781003540830-13

members, friends, and employers. Functionally, this can mean they never get to their personal aspirations, and sometimes rule them out without thinking them through. Addressing self-care needs or actions, people can confuse self-care with being selfish, which they grew up learning not to do. Considering specific situations in context I distinguish between actions for self-made at others' expense and those actions that provide a wellspring of energy and well-being available to be used on others' behalf. The late meditation teacher Sally Kempton (2021) once wrote: "If you want to exercise real, lasting compassion, you need to develop some compassion for yourself."

In their interviews, a number of the MAPS participants mentioned hobbies and volunteer work they enjoyed which seemed to count as self-care along with exercise and healthy eating. I noted, however, that all activities in every category could begin to take over, becoming more obligatory than joyful. Given the reality of 24 hours in a day, and one body, we all have to make choices, without an "all of the above" option. Having sufficient time and space are crucial conditions for self-care, with accompanying shortages of either or both bringing stress. At the same time, self-care can certainly include the pleasure one gains from reciprocal relationships, including a "good talk," regular lunches with friends, and the companionship of a "walking buddy."

Aging

I have two different senses about getting older: (1) I feel like I'm getting kind of older in not so pleasant way – not as vibrant; and (2) I feel older in a good way – internal wisdom embraced a lot more; great in a sense of what you are and what life is about.

Life is boring and I like that. I ignore diabetes as much as I can. Get up in the morning a little creaky, do yoga in bed before I get up. Gravity has hit harder in my face. That special "crepe" look on my arms. I'm much more mellow as the years go by. Everyone is happy about that.

To be all done, there is a sense of sadness realizing that the fertility days are over. That indicates I'm getting old. Run into women in their 80s and 90s and they call me a kid.

Getting older has its pros and cons. I've been reassessing my attitude. I feel some urgency to do certain things in the years I have left. While still healthy, at the same time, I want to enjoy my time, relax now, and have more fun. The wisdom of years of experience is a gift. I like being semi-retired.

I will turn 65 this year. I credit this age, my meditation practice, my counselor, wonderful and challenging family and friends, my myth study group with bringing me to a sense of peace and acceptance than I have ever had in my life.

My general health is essentially the same. Because I do most of the driving now, I drink nothing when we go out. In addition to walking with friend (11 years now) going to the Fit for Life program at the hospital.

I'm taking vitamins now that I'm getting older. Got one of those boxes with days of the week. Used to think those boxes were so stupid.

I feel older and think about moving to a smaller place. I see friends getting older, too, facing health challenges of their own and their spouses. I adore the grandchildren and enjoy life with my husband. We like the quiet.

Life continues to prove interesting. Challenging and rewarding and I love it.

I'm enjoying wisdom that women with age and patience have to "roll with the punches" without sweating the small stuff.

Support

Participants varied in terms of the kinds of support they valued from a partner or spouse. Some kept the details of their menstrual cycles "private" and found questions or assumptions about their cycles by their significant others intrusive. Other participants were the opposite and appreciated the opportunity to share what they were experiencing, being accompanied to medical appointments, and/or their loved one tuning into their changes in health. Feeling supported in their close relationships seemed invaluable, varying from "giving space" to lending a listening ear.

Through the 20 years of the study, I never met formally with family members of the participants, although details could be communicated to me second-hand through the annual updates and family diagrams. Given the dominance of uncertainty at certain junctures of the transition, it would have been natural if loved ones felt equally unsure as to how to best support. (Larson, 2022). Clear communication and a history of having worked through other stressful times played a part in successfully weathering the change, sometimes with input from third-party helpers.

Advocacy

Advocacy, whether on one's own behalf, or for another, generally consists of having a voice in matters important to the persons involved. As such, it may include a number of specific actions, depending on the particular situation. This can include systems advocacy like laws and written or unwritten policies (Center for Excellence in Disabilities West Virginia University, n.d.).

Self-advocacy was central for the MAPS participants going through midlife and the menopause. It could play out at all levels of their lives, with family members, workplaces, and health care providers. There has been much discussion, as well as action, in the areas of patient rights and patient-centered approaches. I think it's fair to say the details as to what these topics represent are worked out and adopted in real time and in context. They have certainly evolved in my lifetime and during my professional work. There has been much written as recommendations to women-as-patients as to how to advocate for themselves to best effect. My own suggestion is first, present yourself as a human being and relate to the human being in the person whose help you are seeking. Problem solving flows more easily from a position of mutual respect, regardless of the distance between views.

Advocacy can include putting into action the suggestions we've covered earlier for good communication, including listening attentively and keeping an open mind. If this is a planned appointment without particular urgency attached, taking time to construct a list of concerns can be helpful to both patient and provider. Expecting to be heard while also remembering the person you're consulting has a schedule and others who need to be heard, too, can help promote a reciprocal interaction. Having supporting documents for questions or concerns can also save time and frame the most important points.

If it is an urgent matter (and even if the appointment is routine), it can be useful to be accompanied by a family member or good friend who can listen, take notes, and perhaps even ask their own questions. Feeling awful physically is a definite barrier to being able to think clearly on the spot and someone who knows the situation well and can maintain their own calm may be an excellent resource managing the incoming information. If decision-making is involved and it's not urgent, there is time to think things over and make a follow-up appointment, possibly even by telehealth. Using the necessary business part of an appointment, including waiting room completion of paperwork, can be an opportunity to breathe and review one's list.

The participants in the MAPS project seemed unusually informed and aware of both their rights and responsibilities when seeking treatment or advice. As a group they were not too intimidated to ask questions and expected clear answers relevant to their situations. In turn, they were forthcoming about reporting the results of these interactions in their annual follow-up interviews. Some contrasted how they typically went about things with how they remembered the women in past generations of their families handling them. They were reluctant to accept recommendations without substantiating reasons for them and saw themselves as having options to seek out second and third opinions if useful to them. When Dr. Freedman suggests "Create your own medical team," he is speaking in wide-ranging terms, conventional as well as complementary medicine, and Eastern approaches as well as Western. In the town where I live, practiced, and in which the majority of the participants resided, there was an assumption that multiple perspectives could be beneficial; an expectation that providers could consult with each other on the participant's behalf; and that feedback along with construction of a plan would be clear and something patients could accept, reject, or modify.

It is essential for people going through major life transitions not to feel alone in the process. It is also important in actualizing one's own agency to approach it as a "matter-of-fact" assumption and not defensively from the get-go. I am very aware that not all women are as fortunate as the participants in this study to have a community from whom they can expect respect. In certain situations, self-advocacy can become social action toward changing unresponsive or limiting systems. Even then, the recommended approach is with confidence in the rightness of the task and not as a victim or angry patron. Speaking openly with listening ears can gain more movement in the long run.

References

Center for Excellence in Disabilities West Virginia University. (n.d.). *Types of advocacy*. https://cedwvu.org/resources/types-of-advocacy/

Freedman, J. (2014). *Stop cancer in its tracks: Your path to mindfulness in healing yourself* (2nd ed.). Create Space Independent Publishing Platform. ISBN-13: 978-15000191542. https://www.mindfulnessinhealing.org

Kempton, S. (2021). *How to cultivate compassion*. https://www.yogajournal.com/lifestyle/balance/relationships/reach-out/

Larson, V. (2022). *How men can support their partners through menopause*. https://greatergood.berkeley.edu/article/item/how_men_can_support_their_partners_through_menopause?utm_source=Greater+Good+Science+Center

Nhat Hanh, T. (2006). *Understanding our mind*. Unified Buddhist Church. Berkeley, CA: Parallax Press. ISBN-13: 978-1888375305

11 For Health Care Providers

When I received my MSW degree in 1975 the Code of Ethics for social work was one page long and filled with what seemed to me to be common sense. By the time I closed my practice in 2013, I'd been licensed for years in my state with the requirement for 3 hours of ethics CEUs every two years. Books, articles, workshops, and lectures were ubiquitous with awful stories about how to not get sued, but not necessarily how to make good contact with clients and be helpful to them (*Standards for the Regulation of Social Work Practice*; professional standards NASW, 1976 & *NASW Code of Ethics,* 1996).

I've enjoyed recently reading work by people in the various helping professions that, again, like the original Code of Ethics, make good sense to me. As I read the bibliographies which accompany the writing, I note some of the ideas that are presented are not a bit "new," but have not really been applied, buried under the dominance of the medical-industrial complex, and again, insurance companies, who to my mind, have turned upside-down meaningful care based on good relationships (Suchman & Matthews, 1988).

What follows in this chapter are considerations for how health care providers can best offer help while also protecting their own humanity.

End of Periods

I think we're done; has gotten sketchy. The last hurrah of the body.

Would just like to never have another period. Pediatrician congratulated me when I started. It was nice to view it positively. It has been a good year. I like the idea I am making some progress. I don't know why I'm supposed to be sad? I enjoyed childbearing but walked away from the marriage – it was not good.

I'm ready, I've bled long enough. Sparse cycles are fine with me.

I appreciate having less investment in products.

There is no HRT with cancer. I use wild yam cream, Dong Quai, no hot flashes anymore. Friend and I went through a variety of products

---

DOI: 10.4324/9781003540830-14

together. I also continued to see complementary medicine specialist. Some hot flashes until aroma therapy took care of the last of those. Sleeping for the first time in 10 years. Wake up at 3 a.m., go to the bathroom, go back to sleep. Wonderful.

Post-hysterectomy is absolutely wonderful. Very much enjoying freedom, lightness of being. Still on 0.05 estrogen patch, no hot flashes. I feel very fortunate. No mood swings, craziness.

So much more freeing to be without period. The first year is kind of life-changing. No chance of ever having a child of my own. Still have a couple of bottles of Midol these many years later – helps with 'hormonal' pain.

There has been a major shift in gravity-shifting south! Dry vagina, very warm, pain on sexual penetration. Husband hates it! Leaking on sneezing and laughing sometimes.

I feel great. Not having any of the hot flashes, insomnia, stress, emotional reactions.

I still have a lot of weight to lose. Doctor says, 'at least not gaining.' I'm 30# heavier than when I married.

Person to Person

Dr. John Launer in *Reflective Practice in Medicine and Multiprofessional Care* (2022) cites a U.S. study showing that "nearly 80% of patients regarded an important attribute of professionalism in doctors as 'preparing before seeing the patient' ... so that we can make eye contact from the moment they enter the room." In his book *Attending: Medicine, Mindfulness, and Humanity*, Dr. Ronald Epstein (2017) carries this idea further:

At its most basic, presence is made visible when the clinician makes good eye contact, responds to patient concerns, and doesn't stand up and leave before the conversation is finished ... when patients say their doctor is "really there," most ... are referring to a quality of being. Presence is a sense of coherence and imperturbability ... listening without interrupting, interpreting, judging, or minimizing ...

The participants in the MAPS study made clear their most useful contacts with health care providers were with people who didn't necessarily have all the answers, but were interested to be helpful on a human-to-human level. Epstein defines the antithesis: "Instead of looking at the patient as a whole person, physicians often view a patient as a sum of the problems that they can recognize, diagnosis and fix." In the latter instance, if this happens routinely with a provider, it can become the reason to leave that situation (Heath, 2014).

Part of "keeping an open mind," even for an expert practitioner, is to be willing to be surprised and curious about "what makes each person tick." As we learn in meditation, the pause, whether between an in-breath and an out-breath, or between exchanges in a conversation, is often an opportunity for clarity, consolidation, and new insights. At the very least it allows for greater calm. I tend to be a person who comes to my annual physical with a list of questions, concerns, or simply a summary of what has occurred in the last year. Wishing to be respectful of my doctor's time I can get speeded up delivering the information and interrupt myself. It is always helpful when she pauses to take in what I have said, looks through the record to see if past history sheds light on a current problem, and/or asks me clarifying questions. Depending on the subject she will then also outline options for management and let me pause to consider them and ask further questions if I have them. We never end an appointment without her asking, "Is there anything else?"

Mindful-Reflective

Launer, whose entire book is focused on "reflective practice," states "reflective practice is *always* possible if you decide it's your main priority." And Epstein emphasizes, "Quieting the mind makes space within the clinician; it promotes openness ... Among doctors who make time for stillness, nearly all feel that the time one makes for contemplative practices-meditation, reflection, awareness-is soon recaptured in increased clarity."

I can say that I lived what these authors were saying when I was in clinical practice. I began training in Bowen Theory in 1982, the same year I opened my private practice after having spent seven years in medical social work in hospitals, dialysis centers, and nursing homes. Eleven years later I began meditating on a daily basis. During my 40 years in a helping profession, the last 30 in private clinical practice, I observed the complexity of daily life had increased as had the baseline stress levels which clients manifested when they arrived for therapy. It was all the more important for me to remain centered and attentive to each person and responsive to their particular dilemmas.

In turn, the skills I used in the clinical work helped taking an observer role as researcher in the MAPS study. No insurance companies were involved. There was no pressure to arrive at a particular outcome, simply to attend with openness as the participants shared their experiences. Many verbalized how useful this was to them to have a setting unconnected to work, home, or family life that allowed them to reflect from year to year on the movement of their bodies (and lives) toward a new reality.

Epstein writes, "'true experts' are mindful and adaptive; they recognize when something's amiss before others do. They observe and respond to context, then switch gears, slowing down and improvising." (Cioffi, 2021; Keshtar et al., 2023).

Productive Partnerships

Both Launer and Epstein emphasize that a mindful and reflective practice both is enhanced by and enhances a collaborative practice. Both practitioners also underline the importance of involving their patients in their own care: not a "do onto" but a "reflect, plan, and decide with." Epstein writes, "Shared decision-making is not only providing information; it is facing uncertainty together." He relates feedback from a patient who attributed her remarkable turn-around in health in large part "to the support she'd received from me and my colleagues." She was specific, include their recognition of her intentions and goals and supporting her as she tried to reclaim her life. She verbalized, "I also like that you're realistic … tell me the truth about my illness, but still give me a reason to hope," that the medical team considered her opinions seriously and said, "I don't know." "At least … I knew you were being honest."

Launer outlines collaborative practice: that it surprises those coming to it new

to find that there is usually a strict ban on giving people advice … people presenting problems need to keep ownership of them and work out the answers for themselves. Presenters want to air their narrative and expose these to the curiosity of others, without being bombarded by suggestions.

Many writing in this field echo his thoughts: "Groups are also good places to learn how to listen attentively, ask good questions, and gain confidence in expressing one's own views." He continues,

presenters (in reflecting teams) nearly always report afterward what a relief it is to speak without interruption, to have an opportunity to clarify the case, and to listen to a range of different perspectives, without having to give an immediate response.

One of the pieces of learning which emerges in collaborative sessions is the realization

there is rarely a single correct way of looking at a clinical case, nor any single correct way of managing it. They can become more at ease with clinical uncertainty, more respectful of their colleagues' opinions, more comfortable about having their own ideas subordinated to the combined expertise of the team, and more compassionate towards complex or challenging patients. (Point of Care Foundation, n.d.)

Similar ideas of embracing complexity, retaining flexibility, and involving all stakeholders in policy and planning are key in achieving creative and useful outcomes. In the real world of the seemingly never-ending demands on time for health care practitioners, Epstein notes, "Elapsed time might be out of a doctor's control to some degree, but perceived time can always be created." He notes as examples of how this happens: sit down, be silent, not rushed. The more professional providers practice this state on a regular basis in quiet time to themselves, the more it can be manifested when consulting with others, whether it be with patients and families, or colleagues (Dugdale, 1999).

Self-Care: Nurturing One's Own Compassion

Working in an adjunct profession along with medical professionals I never aspired to be one of them, taking on that degree of responsibility, the speeded-up schedules, and the multiplicity of requirements. My own profession had its share of pressures, but learning to inject a degree of spaciousness and calm in my day was an accessible and worthy goal. The more pressured one feels, whether seeking or giving help, the more communication suffers, and the feeling of "being alone in a crowd" can intensify. There are certain situations in which a "cure" is not possible, but "care" always is. Dr. Launer quotes a retiring general practitioner, "I'm not a clever doctor, but I am a kind one." And author Anna Quindlen in *Write for your Life* (2022) includes the example of a physician who expresses writing about his experience is his way of reflecting.

In his book, *Attending*, Epstein recounts his own decision to go into medicine was driven by his own illness experiences:

I resolved never to let any patient of mine feel abandoned in this way. I learned in a visceral way that doctors could reduce or worsen a patient's suffering not only through treatments but also by how they behaved and how they chose to share information or not. I envisioned my job as not only to prescribe treatments but also to heal through sharing information, being present, and being kind.

He continues, "I had no idea how difficult that could be." As there has been increasing focus on the mental health of health care providers, programs have been developed to aid the effort to lessen their stress, including ways for health care workers to come together and share stories about their experiences of delivering care. The upshot is that staff can feel more supported and less isolated in their own jobs while better appreciating those of the others (Weisbaum et al., 2023).

References

Cioffi, J. (2021). Situating uncertainty in clinical decision-making. *Academia Letters*, Article 3641. https://doi.org/10.20935/AL3641

Dugdale, D.C., Epstein, R., & Pantilat, S.Z. (1999). Time and the patient-physician relationship. *Journal of General Internal Medicine*. PMCID: PMC1496869

Epstein, R. (2017). *Attending: Medicine, mindfulness, and humanity.* Scribner. ISBN-13: 978-150112121715

Heath, I. (2014). Role of fear in overdiagnosis and overtreatment-an essay by Ione Heath. *The British Medical Journal*. https://doi.org/10.1136/bmj.g6123

Keshtar, L., Madigan, C.D., Ward, A., Ahmed, S., Tanna, V., Rahman, I., Bostock, J., Nockels, K., Wang, W., Gillies, C.L., & Howick, J. (2023). The effect of practitioner empathy on patient satisfaction: A systematic review of randomized trials. Annals *of Internal Medicine*. https://www.acpjournals.org/doi/epdf/10.7326/M23-2168

Launer, J. (2022). *Reflective practice in medicine and multi-professional healthcare.* Boca Raton, FL: CRC Press (and Milton Park, Abingdon). ISBN: 9780367714604

Point of Care Foundation. (n.d.). *Our history and origins.* https://www.pointofcare-foundation.org.uk/about-us/our-history-and-origins/

Quindlen, A. (2022). *Write for your life.* Random House. ASIN:B09BJ7PYQW

Standards for the regulation of social work practice: Professional standards. (1976). Washington, DC National Association of Social Workers. And *NASW Code of Ethics.* (1996). Washington, DC: National Association of Social Workers. https://socialworkers.org

Suchman, A., & Matthews, D. (1988). What makes the patient-doctor relationship therapeutic? Exploring the connexional dimension of medical care. *Annals of Internal Medicine.* https://doi.org/10.7326/0003-4819-108-1-125

Weisbaum, E., Chadi, N., & Young, T. (2023). Improving physician wellness through the Applied Mindfulness Program for Medical Personnel: Findings from a prospective longitudinal study. *CMAJ Open* 11(6).

12 For Researchers

Launching the research project was a venture into the unknown in which I was keenly interested. The kind of study I was undertaking, based on the pillars of Bowen in family systems research and Treloar in menstrual cycle research, was quite different from the projects my dad took on in the natural sciences. Writing his dissertation when I was two years old, moving first into the academic world when I was three, then on to pure research when I was five, and back to academics for the final position of his career when I was nearly eleven, scientific research was a spoken language in our home as long as I can remember.

My own project began 12 years after his death, when he was in his 50s and I was 31. I enjoyed the conversations I was able to have with my mother when I first began reviewing the literature on menopause, and our talks as the project became a reality and progressed. It was a conversation she was used to having, and I felt that taking this path was a homeward journey. At the same time, I saw it as a continuation of my service work, listening to the participants and reinforcing their recordings. Combining the years of my father's research life with my own plus happy exposure to the collaborative emphasis from Bowen theorists to integrate the natural sciences with clinical work, I have observed changes in research emphasis, policy, planning, and funding for over a half century. It is my hope that this final chapter will be useful to other researchers in both the family and menopause fields and demonstrate the overlapping benefits and challenges from research, to the lived lives of the participants, and the efforts of their health care providers. I begin and end with a discussion of complexity.

Updating Our Minds

In *Attending*, Epstein (2017) cites health planners Sholom Glouberman and Brenda Zimmerman describing decisions as "simple, complicated, or complex." He continues, "… in the past 25 years, complexity has skyrocketed" and cautions, "In the face of complexity, the mind strives for efficiency. Too often-to paraphrase H. L. Mencken-we find an answer that is 'clear, simple,

DOI: 10.4324/9781003540830-15

and wrong.'" Launer (2022) in *Reflective Practice in Medicine and Multi-Professional Healthcare* stays with this theme:

> Once you re-orient yourself towards systems thinking, one of the things that you start to notice is now much public policy is guided by what one might call systemic naiveté or even systemic illiteracy. Large-scale initiatives in the public sector nearly always come to grief because someone has made a fundamental error in believing that they can make predictions about how complex human systems will behave. Alongside that error, there is nearly always an even bigger one; the belief that interventions are neutral in themselves and will not involve any costs, risks, or reactions in their own right.

Thankfully, there is a way out of single-minded assumptions to the realization of a multifactorial world that operates in different ways at different levels of organization. In their book, *The Systems View of Life: A Unifying Vision*, co-authors Capra and Luisi (2016) advocate the alternative:

> The emerging new scientific concept of life ... can be seen as part of a broader paradigm shift from a mechanistic to a holistic and ecological world view ... a change from seeing the world as a machine to understanding it as a network.

They and many other scientists and medical professionals working today are becoming clearer the answer is not to throw out meaningful reductionist data and technology nor embrace holism whole-hog, but to generate a larger paradigm which includes both viewpoints and helps the researcher and the health care provider to gain clarity about their focus, the level from which they are currently working, and aiming to explain and/or treat without assuming they have captured the whole. This leaves room for adventure and surprise.

For Launer and Epstein, embracing complexity in practice means to become more comfortable with uncertainty and more committed to addressing each patient within the context of her own world. Epstein states:

> Working with complexity requires what William James called a larger acquaintance with particulars-details of patients and their lives-that often makes us wiser than the possession of abstract formulas, however deep ... [to] know each patient as a person, his genetics and habits, how he responds to illness, whom he lives with and whom he cannot live without, and how his wishes and aspirations affect his decisions ... [to] recognize that every patient is, to some degree, an "n of 1" study, without a control group, and that you have to rely on intuitions and gut feelings.

Launer points out,

> Every intellectual field is born out of a cluster of questions to which answers are either needed or highly desirable ... every field stays alive only to the extent that fresh questions are generated and taken seriously as a driving force in a process of thinking.

My continuing impression from decades of listening to clients and research study participants was they valued being regarded as persons in their own right and consulted about their own observations, views, and aspirations. They didn't expect "miracle cures" for problems so much as respect for their experiences, a discussion of what might be possible, and the hope involved in not being able to predict future outcomes with certainty. Crises arise out of nowhere: as Thich Nhat Hanh would say there are always "causes and conditions" in the present which arose from the past and will in turn have effect into the future, but the only action we can take is here and now (Holst, 2021).

Who Counts?

This section concerns two issues for those researching the menopause transition. First, which populations are included in research, and second, who are the funding sources and which projects do they support.

The year the MAPS project was launched and I also joined the Society for Menstrual Cycle Research, 1991, was a fertile time for menopause research and for considering the issue of proper representation of women participants in that research. Attending my first SMCR conference in June of that year in Seattle, my eyes were opened to the important work being done by multidisciplinary researchers and perspectives which shouldn't have been revolutionary but were.

The Tambrands lecture that year was delivered by Emily Martin (1987) whose book, *The Woman in the Body: A Cultural Analysis of Reproduction*, had been published in that year. Her lecture carried the same title. The SMCR Newsletter which followed the conference reported:

> Emily Martin, professor of anthropology at Johns Hopkins ... presented an analysis of the language used in scientific and medical texts to describe women's reproductive functions. She described how presumably factual descriptions of biological functions serve as metaphors that shape our views of ourselves and others.

Two years later another groundbreaking book was published, *Mismeasure of Woman: Why Women Are Not the Better Sex, the Inferior Sex, or the Opposite Sex* by Carol Tavris (1993). Described at Amazon:

> When "man is the measure of all things," woman is forever trying to measure up ... Tavris unmasks the widespread but invisible custom-pervasive

in the social sciences, medicine, law, and history-of treating men as the normal standard, women as abnormal. Tavris expands our vision of normalcy by illuminating the similarities between women and men and showing that the real differences lie not in gender, but in power, resources, and life experiences.

In what *Vanity Fair* described as "a very personal report," author Gail Sheehy's book *Menopause: The Silent Passage* was first published in 1991 and updated in 2010. I soon realized I had walked into a "hot" field, and was also to benefit personally as these various authors were talking about my own life and experiences which I had never stepped back to consider in these ways. The other papers at the 1991 Conference introduced me to an enthusiastic and supportive community aiming to give women a voice. They had in turn been mentored by other researchers challenging prevailing attitudes and norms, including for one, Patricia A. Kaufert, who had published nearly a decade before "Myth and the menopause," in the July 1982 issue of *Sociology of Health and Illness*. She wrote

> As the use of the word "myth" in the title indicates, this paper is not a discussion of the objective reality of the menopause, but of the representations of the menopause made to women. It focuses on two different perspectives on the menopausal experience, the medical and the feminist. Both the medical profession and the women's health movement claim rights as interpreters to women of their bodies' experience as women. Both groups are anxious that their definitions of menstruation, the processes of childbirth and the menopause should be the ones exclusively accepted by women. Each has developed an elaborate and competing myth of the menopause.

Kaufert concluded: "Neither of these guides to the menopause has been examined for the accuracy with which they describe the experience of most women at their menopause."

Reading this literature, I was set up perfectly for my goal "to study the menopause transition in the context of the participants' lived lives." At the same time, my brief exploration of possible funding sources for conducting such a research study as a sole practitioner/principal investigator without an MD, PhD, or university connection gave me the glimpse of the territory without the means to support it. Not only were women not traditionally the subjects in research which specifically concerned their lives and health, assistance for female researchers and academicians lagged far behind.

In a recent book, *Period: The Real Story of Menstruation*, biological anthropologist Kate Clancy (2023) writes

> I call the particular way we study the menstrual cycle in my lab feminist because of its practice as well as its outcome. Feminist methodology is

deceptively simple: uncover history, look to who holds power, and test the assumptions that tend to underlie it all … Feminist methodology in biology, requires paying special attention to funder, researcher, and subject to whose knowledge is valued, to what research aims get proposed, to what results end up in peer-reviewed literature, and to what ideas and experiences persist even when supposedly rigorous science has ruled them out.

In the same year Clancy's book was published, the field lost noted author and researcher, Evelyn Fox Keller. Her obituary in the *New York Times* (Risen, 2023) described Keller's similar observations:

Dr. Keller trained as a physicist and focused much of her early work on applying mathematical concepts to biology. But as the feminist movement took hold, she began to think critically about how ideas of masculinity and femininity had affected her profession. Like many women in the sciences, she had faced years of disparagement and discrimination, and one of her first efforts was to quantify the effect such a hostile environment had on women-how it held them back, and how it drove many to leave science completely … The problem, Dr. Keller argued, was that gender ideology, and in particular, its emphasis on hard, objective thinking, excluded other modes that might prove equally useful. Feeling, empathy, intuition-these were not necessarily feminine aspects of inquiry, but they all had been excluded from "masculine" scientific methods, while potentially disruptive notions of control and domination has been placed at the center. She called instead for what she called "dynamic objectivity," in which the line between observer and observed was blurred and subjective feelings would be seen as resources-a situation in which, not incidentally, more women might be welcomed into the field.

In a 1986 interview with the *The Boston Globe*, Keller said, "I am not saying that women will do a different kind of science, I am saying when there are more women in science, everybody will be free to do a different kind of science" (Marquard, 2023).

In my own recent reading in systems biology as well as other fields, I am seeing these same perspectives raised by both men and women, and particularly, in scientists from the Western world realizing more readily the short-shrift they have given indigenous medicine and research. In a 2011 issue of the *African Journal of Traditional, Complementary, and Alternative Medicines* the multiauthored article "Traditional Medicine: Past, Present and Future Research and Development Prospects and Integration in the National Health System of Cameroon" the Abstract opens, "Traditional medicine refers to health practices, approaches, knowledge and beliefs incorporating plant, animal and mineral based medicines, spiritual therapies, manual techniques and exercises, applied singularly or in combination to treat, diagnose, and prevent illnesses or maintain well-being (Fokunang, C.N. et al, 2011)."

I have been grateful to have my own consciousness raised, first with Keller's book *A Feeling for the Organism: The Life and Work of Barbara McClintock* (1983) and discussed with Dr. Bowen when I saw it on his bookshelf in one of my personal interviews with him. When I mentioned having read it to him he replied, "Read it again," which I did. Many fine papers from colleagues with the Society for Menstrual Cycle Research through the years have kept me updated on the language and issues of neocolonialism, structural intersectionality, and reproductive and gender justice. As the Earth shrinks with dwindling resources accessed and applied unequally and technology that reaches nearly its every inch, science must open its doors, minds, and purses to its rich diversity.

The Value of Collaboration

An obvious way to support better and more representative research, referenced and reflected by a number of recent authors is useful collaboration. I specify "useful" to indicate something different than people randomly assigned to a required committee, but people from different fields who are challenged and interested to learn from each other, design relevant projects, and both deepen and widen the knowledge base. Clancy in her description of feminist methodology in science asserts it

> requires one to be in conversation with social scientists, historians, and science and technology studies scholars to trace an idea backwards and hear the stories of the people and ideas that were dominant at the time, as well as the views of those who spoke against that dominant thinking.

In *Learning as a Way of Being,* author Peter Vaill (1996) cites Reginald Revans, pioneer of "action learning": "*real* people learn with and from other *real* people by working together in *real* time on *real* problems." In *Resilience Practice: Building Capacity to Absorb Disturbance and Maintain Function* co-authors Walker and Salt (2012) stress the importance of engaging stakeholders to ultimate success in solving real-life problems. I can't stop thinking of Epstein including hospital housekeepers as valuable sources to a medical team trying to understand what might work best for their patients.

I remember my dad talking about a research publication, "I was scooped," as he operated in a research and academic culture of competitive advantage, stacking up publications which led to more and greater grants for the future. He surely had valued colleagues, many of whom we heard from, along with many of his students, of the influence he had in their lives and careers, and in some cases, how they had carried on his work. At the same time, pressures were enormous which I think didn't do his health any favors.

In the Academia Letters column, Alberto Simonetti (2021) wrote on "School and Philosophy": "In the global sharing society, the greatest risk is not sharing knowledge, problems and research … The effort of an interdisciplinary study is long, but the younger generations need a prospective, circular, inter-dynamic."

In an article in *Nature*, "Try a Touch of Intellectual Humility," writer Jane Palmer (2023) summarized "Being open to the limitations of their knowledge can help researchers to foster interdisciplinary and cross-cultural collaborations." She described the situation of Ike de la Pena, a research pharmacologist in Loma Linda University visiting his home country, the Philippines, as part of its Balik ("returning") Scientist Program, and meeting with local researchers to explore potential areas for collaboration. Encountering a lack of energy in a Zoom meeting, "he did the opposite of taking control. He exercised humility." Explaining he was there "not to impose his ideas or create change, but to learn," "the atmosphere in the meeting changed … Everybody began just smiling and freely sharing their ideas."

That description to me is reminiscent of the atmosphere I so valued in the Research Workshops at Georgetown around the turn of the last century. Palmer quoted Michael Lynch, a philosopher at the University of Connecticut, "Somebody who has intellectual humility understands that they aren't going to simply climb on top of a mountain of knowledge themselves. They recognize it is going to take some help." She added the view of Tenelle Porter, a psychologist at Rowan University in Glassboro, NJ, "Intellectual humility can really help us listen to those who don't have the same ways of knowing as we do or those with a different expertise."

Dr. Dan Siegel https://drdansiegel.com/interpersonal-neurobiology/n.d. whose work focuses on "interpersonal neurobiology" states: "This interdisciplinary approach invites all branches of science and other ways of knowing to come together and find the common principles from within their disparate approaches to understanding human experience." I understand this to mean the richness of true collaboration is expressed in the container of mutual respect for difference. To deal with the complex world the tools are not found in endless homogeneity, but expansive and dynamic diversity.

Self-care: Managing Time and Purpose

In "Research in the speed of light? A brief reflection on contemporary academic production," Clarissa Campo (2021) described the dilemma of managing both time and purpose to the advancement of science. She stated:

> As someone who always had a considerable degree of difficulty coping with the tons of information we receive on a daily basis, while listening to how Darwin came to write his seminal work, it was how time was a

key factor for his achievements that provoked me the most. The time to observe, investigate, and reflect; and the time to essentially enjoy what he was doing and enjoy life while he was doing it … it is worth questioning whether the possibilities offered by recent technologies to produce more have deprived us of precious time to produce better. The idea here is not to turn back time, nor that it is bad that we are all connected in real-time. Advances in communication technologies and the possibilities contained in being able to easily reach and exchange information with people around the globe, as we know, have innumerable advantages. My question refers to how we have been producing, to what end, and at what costs.… when we engage and reinforce frantic dynamics, aren't we reproducing some of the oppressive logics that many of us, myself included, strongly refute?

As I read her letter, I thought of my dad complaining (allegedly jokingly, but for real) that he didn't have time to make any progress because he was always writing progress reports. I thought of my client on faculty at university and raising two children, who was feeling overloaded in all aspects of her life. Her specific question in a clinical session was the invitation to serve on yet another committee, which was (allegedly) a compliment and a route to add to her resume, but for which she literally had no time. I shared that when my daughter was a toddler and I was invited to serve on various community boards, I had finally learned to express gratitude along with a refusal which indicated I take service seriously and would not be able to serve to the best of my ability given my other obligations. No one ever argued with me and often the conversation ended with the idea if circumstances changed, I could be considered again. My client's eyes opened with the realization she had never thought of this option. Afterward, she called me and said, "It worked!"

I hope it is clear that I have included self-care in every section of these recommendations. I believe that compassion is not only essential for health, well-being, and rewarding relationships but also fundamental for transacting a complex, ever-speedy world. At some point we need to recognize some of our deadlines and the ever-constant striving are self-imposed and not helpful to ourselves, our work, or those with whom or on behalf of whom we are interacting. Increasingly, reports are written with the testimony of the spaciousness present in stopping to take a breath, a walk in nature, or enjoy a smile with a stranger. Do research ideas emerge from those activities? Absolutely! And often with greater clarity of what avenues would produce the best, most interesting, or most worthy result. When we allow ourselves to live lives of purpose and meaning with ample space for reflection and invention, we serve as models to our fellow midlife friends, or children, or research associates. Those opportunities will not be handed to us. We must design, construct, and follow through.

> **After Menopause**
>
> Awesome; quite pleased to be through the mess and the distress.
>
> No sadness really, it was time.
>
> I think we'll be a great group of oldsters.
>
> Blank book – don't even think about it. No symptoms to look at. Life marches along. I don't have to worry when go out backpacking, long trip, where I am in cycle.
>
> I have lots of energy – menopausal zest! Occasional difficulty falling or staying asleep.
>
> Haven't missed it, haven't missed the pain. Similar to childbirth. Time or two had what resembled a menstrual cramp. I have much greater appreciation of women the older I get.
>
> I've adjusted happily to not having periods and I no longer notice the disconcerting feeling that I am about to start my period as I did for several years. My mood seems more consistent in general, although I still get depressed at times. For my temperature sensitivity, I wear layers and adjust the thermostat in my house a lot.
>
> I listen to all the medical programs as much as I can. I can't say I am in postmenopausal zest, but my energy is much better. My friend and I continue to hike up to 15 miles although have slowed down some.
>
> It's nice to not have your period, but not nice to not have those elements in your body that create the period. I had an easy period all my life. Now skin and hair are drier and I can't get the weight off.
>
> Definitely experiencing postmenopausal zest now. I feel a curse has been lifted; I never in my early years thought of it being a curse.
>
> Menopause signifies a new time in my life, helping me realize what is really important to me and wondering how much time I have left on this planet.
>
> I basically am enjoying my postmenopause life, marriage, and health, feeling blessed and more at peace with myself than I've ever been. The main anxiety is knowing this can't last forever.
>
> Menopause is so long ago.

References

Campo, C. (2021). Research in the speed of light? A brief reflection on contemporary academic production. *Academic Letters*, Article 357. https://doi.org/10.20935/AL357

Capra, F. & Luisi, P. (2016). *The systems view of life: A unifying vision.* Cambridge University Press reprint edition. ASIN: 1316616436 ISBN-13: 978-1316616437.

Clancy, K. (2023). *Period: The real story of menstruation.* Princeton University Press. ISBN-13: 978-0691191317.

Epstein, R. (2017). *Attending: Medicine, mindfulness, and humanity.* Scribner. ISBN-13: 978-150112121715.

Fokunang, et al, *Afr J Tradit Complement Altern Med* (2011) 8(3): 284–295.

Holst, M. (2021). To be is to inter-be: Thich Nhat Hanh on interdependent arising. *Journal of World Philosophies* 6 (winter 2021):17–30.

Kaufert, P. (1982). Myth and menopause. *Sociology of Health and Illness* 4(2): 141–166.

Keller, E. (1983). *A feeling for the organism: The life and work of Barbara McClintock.* New York: W.H. Freeman and Company.

Launer, J. (2022). *Reflective practice in medicine and multi-professional healthcare.* Boca Raton, FL: CRC Press (and Milton Park, Abingdon). ISBN: 9780367714604.

Martin, E. (1987). *The woman in the body: A cultural analysis of reproduction.* Beacon Press. ISBN-13: 978-0807046043.

Marquard, B. (2023). Evelyn Fox Keller, MIT professor emerita who challenged gender bias in science, dies at 87. https://www.bostonglobe.com.

Palmer, J. (2023). Try a touch of intellectual humility. *Nature* 6225.

Risen, C. (2023). Evelyn Fox Keller, who turned a feminist lens on science. *NYTimes* https://www.nytimes.com>2023/09/30.

Sheehy, G. (2010). *The silent passage* (6th ed.) Gallery Books.ISBN: 978-1451607420.

Siegel, D. website. *An introduction to interpersonal neurobiology.* https://drdansiegel.com/interpersonal-neurobiology

Simonetti, A. (2021). School and philosophy. *Academic Letters*, Article 1474.

Tavris, C. (1993). *The mismeasure of women.* Touchstone. ISBN-13: 978-0671797492.

Vaill, P. (1996). *Learning as way of being: Strategies for survival in a world of permanent white water.* San Francisco, CA: Jossey-Bass, Inc. ISBN-13: 978-0787902469.

Walker, B. & Salt, D. (2012). *Resilience practice: Building capacity to absorb disturbance and maintain function.* Island Press. ISBN: 978-1597268011.

Index

For Product Safety Concerns and Information please contact our EU
representative GPSR@taylorandfrancis.com
Taylor & Francis Verlag GmbH, Kaufingerstraße 24, 80331 München, Germany